PERIODS AREN'T MEANT TO BLOODY HURT

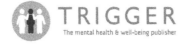

TRIGGER

The mental health & well-being publisher

PERIODS AREN'T MEANT TO BLOODY HURT

GEMMA BARRY

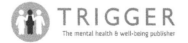

TRIGGER
The mental health & well-being publisher

Published in 2023 by Trigger Publishing
An imprint of Shaw Callaghan Ltd

UK Office
The Stanley Building
7 Pancras Square
Kings Cross
London N1C 4AG

US Office
On Point Executive Center, Inc
3030 N Rocky Point Drive W
Suite 150
Tampa, FL 33607
www.triggerhub.org

A CIP catalogue record for this book is available upon request from the British Library
ISBN: 978-1-83796-294-5
Ebook ISBN: 978-1-83796-295-2

I'd like to dedicate this book to Lizzie –
One of the best humans I know x

CONTENTS

Introduction   ix

Part 1: Why Periods Hurt   **1**
1   A Period Drama   3
2   The Endocrine System:
        Getting to Know Your Hormones   15
3   A Deep Dive into Hormones   25
4   Charting Your Cycle   31
5   Understanding PMS   45
6   Unpacking Red Flags   53
7   Specific Conditions   65
8   Being Seen and Heard   77
9   A Quick History of Synthetic Hormones   89

Part 2: What You Can Do About It   **99**
10   Nutrition   101
11   Oestrogen Dominance   123
12   Plants! As Medicine?   141
13   Exercise   153
14   I Can't Stress This Enough   169
15   Your Frame of Mind   185
16   Period Stigma and Shame   205

Part 3: Heading into Menopause   **213**
17   The Perimenopause: Welcome to Limbo Land   215
18   Menopause: The Cloak of Invisibility Sequins   229

The Final Round-up   241
The Well Woman Project   243
Useful Resources   245
Acknowledgements   247
References   249

INTRODUCTION

If your actions create a legacy that inspires others to dream more, learn more, do more and become more, then you are an excellent leader.

Dolly Parton

Hi – I'm Gemma Barry, and I worked as a nurse for 15 years in busy London hospitals and have always had a keen interest in health. I left nursing to explore the holistic side of health, which led me to train as a reflexologist and massage therapist, and to set up my own business, which I have been running for over a decade. Since being diagnosed with endometriosis and adenomyosis seven years ago, I retrained as a herbalist, mindfulness practitioner and Mizan therapist (Mizan is a specific pelvic and abdominal massage therapy), and have become a complete geek about hormonal and period health. This has all led me on a bit of a journey, discovering the many holes we have had in our education and understanding of our own bodies. My mission is to set that straight.

What else do you need to know? I have blue or green hair, an affection for the 80s, I LOVE sequins – they can turn a bad day right around – and my wardrobe looks like a disco ball. I'm a stand-up comedian and wrote a one-woman show called *Flaps of Steel*. I love to garden, I have a husband called Mark and a dog called Indie, and they both snore. I like sewing, second-hand clothes and belly laughs that make you practise using your pelvic floor muscles. Although I used to be a nurse, I don't miss it, but I do miss sorting out a manky wound. I'm also learning magic and I have a fab selection of colourful shoes.

A NEW WAY

The more I learned about my conditions and the treatments available, the more I realised there is a whole other world in looking after our health that falls outside of the mainstream consciousness. I had been to the doctors about my menstrual health problems, and I was given the usual three-pronged treatment: painkillers, hormones and anti-depressants.

This book is my way to help you challenge this conventional approach and give you all the information you need to manage your health another way.

Pain has been normalised when it comes to period health – it is so enmeshed in our experience. No one sees it as a major problem that we just carry on regardless, and this is having detrimental effects on our everyday lives. Dealing with pain and all the other fanny admin that comes with feral periods and raging hormones means that all facets of our lives get affected, our well-being plummets, and we start to wonder if we are making this up.

I want you to be your own advocate. I will give you practical tips – things you can use to become your own detective about your hormonal health and, above all else, make you realise that periods aren't meant to bloody hurt, and it's a problem if they do!

Since I straddle both worlds, I have a wealth of understanding and experience in both the traditional medical model and the holistic model. My aim is to give you all the information you need to help you steer yourself through your health choices in ways we are not always shown.

I have included some history about how we are in the place we find ourselves with our health and education – thanks, patriarchy!

It is so important to have an understanding of where this stems from so that you can go on to educate yourself on these matters and also support and pass this on to future generations.

We are slowly waking up to the importance of our bodies and what they are about, but we still have a long way to go. Science still generally shrugs its shoulders and says, 'Sorry we didn't include women in this study because their bodies are too complicated.' Women make up 50% of the people on the planet, and we should have a better representation of our bodies in science and education. Can you think of a time you were taught about your cervical secretions?! This is why we worry that there is something wrong with us!

I would also like to take this moment to acknowledge that **not all women have periods**. Non-binary and trans folk also need help in being able to address menstrual health matters in a safe and non-judgmental way. As an intersectional feminist, I acknowledge and support them throughout this book. I have been interchangeable with my language, but I know the issues I write about in here don't just affect biological women. I hope that if you are reading this as a trans or non-binary person, you can get something out of it. I am always open and willing to talk through ways in which I can support this community better.

WHY I WROTE THIS BOOK

This book has been an ember and then a fire, and I hope that I pass that light to you, and you can go forth with more light and power to make yourself heard in this very noisy world of ours.

I wrote this book because over ten years ago I collapsed in a pub toilet while I was out with my husband, and it's something I never want to happen to me again. Being a nurse, having the general public trying to diagnose me and slapping me around the face petrified me – I thought I was going to have surgery right there on the tiled floor. It was quite the drama in the pub for a little bit. Mark missed the rugby, and I got carted off to A&E.

When they got me into the department, I heard the paramedic say, 'I don't think she is in as much pain as she says she is', but was surprised to see I had drained the gas and air machine, had two doses of morphine and some diclofenac, and was still writhing around in pain.

I was asked if I was pregnant a billion times, and they ruled out appendicitis because it was the wrong side. I had a scan, as they thought it was kidney stones, although I didn't pass any nor did they see any on the scan. Eventually, the pain subsided and I was discharged home with no follow-up – just told to see my GP if it happened again and, oh, drink plenty of water.

I had always had pretty ropey periods. I started on the pill when I was 16 to try to even them out, but it didn't really help. I remember more than once being doubled over in pain when I had my period, but I was told that was just how it was, so that's what I believed.

I went to my doctor numerous times with pelvic pain and sex being uncomfortable. They told me to take painkillers, relax more when having sex, and as I was on the pill, not much more could happen.

I had to stop taking the pill a few years later due to migraines, and this was the first time I had seen my natural cycle in a long time. It was wild and all over the place – I never knew when I was going to get a period, and always had to carry emergency supplies and just pray to the blood goddess that I didn't erupt and leave a mark on the seat of the train.

Then I collapsed in the pub and was told I had kidney stones, which I believed for years with all the griping pains I had, so I would drink more water – I had amazing skin, I tell ya! There were many times I would come over feeling really sick, sweaty and unable to stand. I would need to just lie on the floor, I would feel faint and horrendous, but I never passed out. It would ease off and I'd think, 'There goes another bloody stone.'

Then, about seven years ago, I passed out again at home, coming round to the dog licking my face. I had fainted while on the toilet. The pain was unbelievable. I slowly made my way to the bed and rang Mark to come home because I felt awful. I just thought it was another bad flare up of stones, but when he came home and saw me, off to hospital we went. Thankfully, they could see I was in serious amounts of pain, and I got given lots of nice drugs that knocked me out a treat. I slept for about two hours straight, having been rocking on all fours for hours – it looked like I was in labour. They booked me for a CT scan, and it turned out I had an ovarian cyst the size of a cantaloupe hanging off one of my ovaries. I needed surgery ASAP because this thing was twisting my ovary, and it was at risk of bursting.

I walked around for the next few weeks like I had a bomb in my belly. I couldn't have sex or do any other physical activity – I was to sit down and do nothing. When I went for my consultation for the surgery, my consultant said she would just chop off the ovary because I didn't want children, so it didn't matter to lose one. I made it quite clear that I wanted to keep my ovary, regardless on my standpoint of having kids – I was born with two and I wanted to keep them both!

The surgery went well. Persephone (as I named my cyst) had teeth and hair and fingernails in her – a mutant! It was also discovered I had quite advanced endometriosis, and I was told I would need to start taking hormones straight away, as it was the only way to deal with this. I explained that I couldn't take the combined pill because it triggered migraines, and that I had tried the progesterone-only version and that had also given me awful headaches that didn't budge. My consultant commented that I was a sensitive flower, and I asked her if I could help myself with any other route. She said no, but had heard yoga was helpful. She also said that if I didn't follow her way of doing things, I would be back in her office in ten years' time begging for a hysterectomy.

My follow-up letter arrived and it said I had had an oophorectomy (removal of ovary). I hopped on the phone to the huffy secretary who said, no, that hadn't actually happened, and they would send another letter. The second letter arrived and said the same thing. I rang again and said I wanted a scan – I'd lost faith in their record-keeping and wanted to see that ovary for myself.

Funny how things turn out, because in doing that (and confirming my ovary was still there), I also found out I have adenomyosis (see page 68) and fibroids. It wasn't the news I necessarily wanted but I felt like I had all the facts now. I was discharged from their care, and I haven't seen a health professional since. I have routine blood tests and I request ultrasound scans to keep an eye on things but, other than that, I go by how my body feels and what my period is doing.

I share this story and its comedy of errors because I know I'm not alone, and I talk a lot about how the medical system fails women. It failed me, I was misdiagnosed, not heard, not listened to, patronised, belittled and disregarded. I, myself, am a health professional, so I have a head start on how the system works, and I was still left wanting.

I had already started to take matters into my own hands before all of this and I was confident that I could, and would, find a way through this that didn't involve relying on medication my body couldn't handle.

One of the first things I changed was my period products. I switched from commercial ones to a menstrual cup and reusable pads. My cycle changed – it started to regulate, which was something I had never experienced before. In my personal experience, I came to learn a lot about what was in our period products that could have accounted for what I had experienced. This encouraged me to get curious with more aspects of my hormonal health. I changed up my diet bit by bit, reducing inflammation in my body. I read everything I could get my hands on about all the things that were hanging around inside me. I did specialist pelvic massage, I started to sort through my emotional shit, I used herbs, I used supplements, I rested and, slowly but surely, I started to feel a lot better. I'll cover all of this in Part 2.

MY MISSION

I don't say I cured my endo, adeno and fibroids, but I have healed the symptoms that they were giving me. I don't have irregular periods anymore, and I don't have pain. My periods are still a bit heavy, but I wouldn't really expect anything else on that score, really. I put my body first in healing what it needed to heal.

I also realised I had a niche set of skills in being a nurse who understood medical jargon and had 15 years' experience in a wide range of fields, but also being a massage therapist, mindfulness practitioner, herbalist, doula, hypnobirthing teacher, reflexologist and reiki practitioner. So, I bundled them all up and started The Well Woman Project, the business I founded to share my knowledge and help other women with their hormonal health.

In the years I have been running it, I have helped educate and empower women to have a better understanding of their periods and bodies. I even wrote a one woman show, *Flaps of Steel*, which is an edutainment dive into periods, vaginas and how our health system was shaped.

Every time I would mention that periods didn't have to hurt, I would get quite a bit of stick for it, with comments ranging from being told that I didn't know what I was talking about to being called a quack. It's a tough gig when you think differently sometimes, but as they say, the haters gonna hate, and here I am having written a book with the exact statement that caused such a fuss.

I have worked with a wide and varied amount of people with endo, adeno, PMDD, heavy bleeds, painful bleeds, fatigue, feral moods and more. They get a hold of me feeling totally hopeless, feeling like they are going mad, and I offer them hope, something they haven't felt in a very long time. Everyone I have worked with has had positive transformations in so many different ways, and I am forever humbled by this – you teach me so much!

For us to have better autonomy and body literacy, things need to shift at the ground level. The more we talk and the more we open up about our experiences, the more we complain and don't silence ourselves against a system never designed for our bodies in the first place, the more people will have to take notice. Not talking about periods and hormones plays directly into the patriarchy's hands. We aren't and never were broken, inferior, a mangled version of a man's body or hysterical – these are all labels given to us by those that had no idea, and the legacy has lasted a very long time.

I share my personal story because I know I'm not alone with the kerfuffle I experienced – but just because it happens a lot doesn't make it right.

Your period is not meant to bring you to your knees every month, it isn't meant to be such a fiasco that you can't go about your normal activities of daily living. If you are impacted that much, something isn't right.

ABOUT THIS BOOK

This book is presented in three parts. Part 1 is an in-depth exploration as to why your periods might be hurting you and how you can investigate this further. We take a look at your body and particularly your hormones, which are the key to so much when trying to fix troublesome periods. I talk about the importance of charting your cycle – what this means and how it improves body literacy – and how we need better advocacy in dealing with the medical profession concerning our menstrual health.

Part 2 moves on to look at what we can do about painful periods and related conditions. I encourage a holistic approach and explore how nutrition, herbs, exercise and your frame of mind can all not only support your menstrual health, and health in general, but can achieve transformative results in terms of your periods.

And finally, Part 3 takes a look at what's to come once your periods stop, with chapters on the perimenopause and menopause itself. Rather than something to be approached with fear and dread, we consider your post-period future and reframe it as a positive transition to a new chapter.

I have enjoyed decanting my brain into these pages for you. I really hope that you find it helpful, have a few laughs and above all, you gain more insight into your body and the things you can do to improve your health. Let's dive in.

PART 1

WHY PERIODS HURT

In order to trust your body as a guide, the first step is to understand it.

Deepak Chopra

I always find it helpful to start with the foundation and build upon it. Hormonal health is a massive topic, and all too often we start trying to fix things at a surface level without knowing what underpins it.

It's one thing to say our hormones are on the wonk, but when we start to understand what our hormones are and then look at the intricate relationship hormones have with each other, it begins to paint a clearer picture.

I also think it helps if you are anything like me and want to know why things are the way they are. I feel all too often we are given the narrative that it is just the way things are when, really, we do have a lot more control over those things than we may believe we have.

CHAPTER 1

A PERIOD DRAMA

Improving menstrual health in schoolgirls can lead to long-lasting effects on women's overall education, health and well-being.

Helen Weiss

Honestly, if you read this section and think, 'Why didn't I know this?' – I feel you. It's a testament to the lack of education we have had, so don't sweat it; you will know it now, and that is the main thing. Aspects of our periods that aren't normal have been normalised over time, so we find ourselves accepting painful periods, which we should not be. This leads us to struggle in silence with heavy, painful periods or feral PMT (premenstrual tension), and becomes something most women become accustomed to. Pain is, and never will be, a 'normal' experience in your body.

I don't like averages or 'norms', because as I am keenly aware, most people sit outside of them – and that is fabulous. However, when it comes to periods and hormones, we do need some benchmarks so we can tell when ours might be going into uncharted territory. Throughout this chapter – and book – I have given averages and 'norms', but if your norms sit outside of them and they don't give you any bother, then do bear that in mind.

Right, let's jump in and unpack this bit by bit so you pop out the other end of this chapter fully informed. Ready? Let's be having you, then…

A PERIOD UNPACKED

Let me be absolutely crystal clear with you, periods should **NOT** hurt, and they should **NOT** be excessively heavy. We will unpack this further as we proceed in this book, but for the love of Goddess, please, if you are experiencing either – or both – stop putting up with it and get it investigated because it is **NOT** normal.

Your cycle is the continuous motion of change in your body, literally no two days are the same. It's like being in a continuous state of redecorating: you are either in the exciting stage of faffing around with soft furnishings and colours or tearing it all down to start again. It's always in a state of flux – which is normal, by the way – hence it's called a cycle. The aim of the game is not to turn that cycle into a line, but to turn it into something that

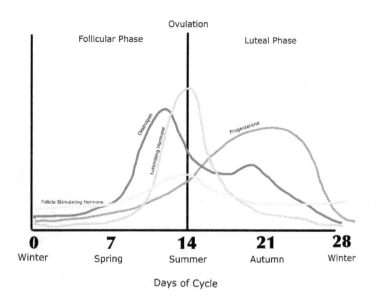

Days of Cycle

flows like a beautiful piece of music with no awful, improvised jazz notes spiking through and making your ears bleed. Apologies to anyone who is a jazz fan but, seriously, how do you listen to that?!

Your period is the beginning of your menstrual cycle, and the first day of your bleed is Day 1. It is one part of the whole cycle, and it's where we can learn a lot about our overall health, but there is also a lot to learn from the rest of the cycle. Think of your period as being a production on stage, while the rest of the time in your cycle, things are going on behind the scenes, all of which impact the final performance.

There is so much going on during your cycle, it's best digested by being broken down into phases. If you find this next bit a lot, just be thankful your body takes care of it without you having to organise it each month – that'd be one hell of an event to be planning all the time!

Everyone has different cycle lengths – they are usually between 21 and 35 days. The average is around 28 days, but this isn't the gold standard. As long as you have the same number, give or take a day or two every month, you have a happy cycle. What governs the timing of your period and length of your overall cycle is down to three things:

1. **The follicular phase (TFP)** – the first half of your cycle, which can last 7–21 days
2. **Ovulation (O)** – happens in the middle of your cycle and lasts 1 day
3. **The luteal phase (TLP)** – the second half of your cycle, which lasts 12–14 days (but no more that 14 days as that is the maximum life span of the corpus luteum, see page 7)

TFP + O + TLP = the length of your cycle. You can work this out retrospectively counting back through your dates, or if you use a tracker app, it will have that info. This is important knowledge for you if you want to start working with your cycle.

THE FOLLICULAR PHASE

The follicular stimulating hormone is released from the pituitary gland and does what it says on the tin – it stimulates your follicles to grow and release oestrogen. The oestrogen you produce through your follicles is called oestradiol, and it stimulates the uterine lining to thicken and grow. As you head towards ovulation, oestrogen peaks, and then it starts to dip after ovulation.

FOLLICLES

These are the small sacs inside your ovaries that are in the making long before an egg ever pops out of them. The health of your follicles is indicative of the periods and symptoms you might be experiencing. It's really important to note that when working with your period and cycle, you are technically always working in the past. The period you have now is telling you how the last three months have gone because it takes 100 days for your follicle to mature enough to think about popping eggs out of it. This means the care you take of yourself now will be seen in the periods of your future. It's a bit mind-bendy, I grant you, but suffice it to say working with your period isn't a quick-fix project – it can and often does take some time.

OVULATION

There is no 'maybe' when it comes to ovulation – you either do or you don't! As the follicles jostle to the finish line, one, or rarely two (this is how non-identical twins happen), burst forth with an egg, triggered by the luteinising hormone from the pituitary gland.

The egg busting out of the follicle happens in seconds, but you can have hours of the follicles swelling like balloons until one goes *pop*. This is why some can notice it and feel some twinges.

Once that egg has broken free, you will either see a period in two weeks' time, or you will be pregnant. It's impossible to ovulate and not see a period – unless you are preggo.

THE LUTEAL PHASE

Once the egg has left its follicle home, that follicle then morphs itself into an endocrine gland called the corpus luteum, which secretes progesterone. This is no mean feat; in just 24 hours it goes from a ruptured follicle to a 4cm endocrine gland. In terms of the miracles the body can perform, this is up there, believe me.

Ovulation is so important because it's how we form the corpus luteum, and without that we wouldn't be producing progesterone. The progesterone is the yin to the oestrogen's yang – they are night and day to each other. Progesterone has a calming effect on the nervous system, whereas oestrogen stimulates it.

If you are pregnant, the corpus luteum supports the pregnancy for the first three months until the placenta takes over. If you aren't pregnant, it will be reabsorbed back into your body. It can only survive a maximum of 14 days, so this means your luteal phase can only be 12–14 days long. Progesterone builds through this part of your cycle, peaking in the middle, and then tails off towards your period, which indicates to the uterus to contract and dance the funky chicken to clear its lining for the next DIY project.

MEASURING YOUR PROGESTERONE

Measuring hormones with blood tests can be tricky at the best of times, but progesterone can be a real slippery customer. The levels in your body can fluctuate within a space of just 90 minutes! To test it you need to be in the middle of your luteal phase – it is commonly known as 'day 21 progesterone', but that is only good if you have a 28-day cycle. To measure effectively, you will need to adapt this day accordingly to your cycle length. If you have an irregular cycle, it can be a bit of a stab in the dark at best, but you will need to aim to do it about a week out from your period.

THE BIG P

If all is well with your hormones and you have had adequate amounts of everything, and your follicle health is good, your period should arrive with little to no fanfare. It should be a balanced flow with no PMT, pain, flooding, large clots, etc. I see you rolling your eyes at me because I know very well that is NOT the norm that most experience and that, my friends, breaks my heart.

NOT GETTING THE BIG P

If you don't get a period and you aren't pregnant, then this is called an *anovulatory period*. This means you didn't go through all the stages above; your body didn't ovulate and there was no corpus luteum, progesterone or luteal phase. Sometimes, you can still bleed, but it isn't a 'true' period and the periods tend to be irregular.

Since the follicles secrete oestrogen, the lining of the uterus will thicken and thicken until eventually it falls away and you bleed. So how do you know you haven't ovulated? This is where charting comes in. Charting simply means making daily observations about your cycle, over several months or on an ongoing basis, so you can start to recognise patterns and better understand your own body and menstrual health. In particular, taking your basal body temperature is a good indication of ovulation – I will talk more about this later.

However, even without charting, there will be signs, such as:

- Your periods will often be really random and all over the shop.
- Usually there is some spotting before and after.
- Your periods just won't feel the same as they normally do.

This type of bleed is very common during your perimenopause and with PCOS (polycystic ovary syndrome), and it is also always worth getting your thyroid levels checked if this is happening.

Let's look at the cycle more closely, specifically at some red flags that should not be welcome around the table.

RED FLAGS

We have got to a point that we are unable to question the feralness of our periods because it has become so normal for them to be awful that we don't realise just how bad things are. Our poor period health is basically hiding in plain sight. Even when we do go to seek help, more often than not we are told all is normal and it is to be expected, or other areas of the body are looked at rather than addressing the main problem we have. This repeated gaslighting has bred a culture of dysfunction and has led to us not trusting our bodies and seeking external band-aid fixes.

I know that for a lot of you, going to your doctor with these kinds of problems will lead you to coming away with a prescription for synthetic hormones, painkillers or anti-depressants – if it's a really bad day, you might score the hat-trick and get all three.

Again, I will unpack this later but, for now, let's look at what a period should **NOT** be like.

Here is a list of some of the more common red flags that sometimes get ignored, tolerated or normalised. I will contextualise this by saying that we should always be looking for patterns that the symptoms of our cycle and period give us. Occasionally, we might get blips – one of the red flags turns up for a one-off appearance and is never seen again. Charting your period and cycle allows you to see patterns forming and be ahead of the game rather than being pushed about by it all.

YOUR PERIOD SHOULD NOT LOOK LIKE...

- Pain and the use of over-the-counter pain relief – needing to medicate your period 'to get through it' every month, without which you wouldn't be able to function
- Needing to change your period product every hour or less, and it's soaked and perhaps even leaking
- Needing to wear several types of period products to go about your daily business because you leak through everything
- Significant bleeding at night that interrupts your sleep
- A period that lasts for more than seven days
- Significant mood disruptions
- Bleeding outside of your period (sometimes ovulation spotting can happen and that's OK)
- An offensive odour
- No period at all and you aren't pregnant
- Irregular periods
- Changes to your cycle/period – these might take a while to show and is why I advocate charting your cycle, so you

can see these patterns happening before they are worse than they need to be

• Painful sex – sex should never, ever be painful

If you have ticked off one or more things on that list, then you need to know these are not normal functions of having periods and they signify that something isn't right.

I BLEED BUT I DON'T DIE

Menstruation, or your period, is the time you are actively bleeding. On 'average' it can last anywhere from 2–7 days, and it is usual to lose anywhere from 25–80mls of blood – the 'average' being around 50mls. Ideally, a period has an even flow and a rhythm to it, and it *absolutely shouldn't bring you to your knees*. Again, and I'll keep saying this, unless you document your cycle, somehow you won't see or notice the more subtle things.

This is an example of a bog-standard flow:

• Day 1: Bleeding starts, continuous but fairly light
• Day 2: Heavier bleeding
• Day 3: Heavier bleeding
• Day 4: Lighter bleeding
• Day 5: Lighter bleeding / spotting / stops

The length of your period will determine how that looks for you, but ideally you don't have more than two days of heavy bleeding – it is a red flag if you do. It is also important to have a period and, like Goldilocks, it should be just right – too short and it's showing problems, too long and it's showing problems.

Shorter and lighter periods are often thought of as the dream, but they are also indicative of hormonal imbalance, and to not have them at all is of concern. Obviously, pregnancy is a perfectly good reason as to why they might have stopped, but there are a lot of other reasons that aren't so great – such as being underweight or over-stressed, or over-exercising. Our bodies won't have the reserves to actually make a period if they don't have the sufficient nutrients to do so. If periods aren't seen for months at a time, this could indicate PCOS. It can also be indicative of the perimenopause (see page 215).

Sometimes, we can have just the mother of all periods and then normal service resumes. Keep a note, though, because one-offs don't spell disaster, but if they start to become a thing then this is a change, and it needs to be investigated.

Periods that go on for a week or two are also not a wonderful place to be. Underlying health conditions can make this happen, such as hormonal imbalances, fibroids, endometriosis or adenomyosis. Taking tranexamic acid, which is often prescribed, is all very well, but it won't get to the bottom of why periods are heavy in the first place. Neither will taking synthetic hormones.

BLOODY MARVELLOUS

To give you an idea of how much blood you are losing, here are some numbers. A regular tampon/pad holds approximately 5mls; a super tampon/pad holds approximately 10mls. Using menstrual cups will give you more accuracy, and reusable pads may well hold a bit more. If you aren't saturating the whole product, then you need to adjust accordingly.

Calculating blood loss gives you more of an idea about your flow. I have worked with lots of women who were blissfully unaware their flow was as heavy as it was, just thinking it was the norm – it isn't. This is why talking about it is so important because we get to realise our lived experiences aren't the same as everyone else's, and that we are most likely putting up with shitty periods when we don't need to. I would go so far as to say that periods are the one area of our lives where we really want to be comparing notes with others because it is illuminating and so helpful.

So, if your period is somewhere in the middle of 25–80mls, that will be approximately ten regular tampons/pads or five super-soakers. Your flow should ease off at night, so you shouldn't be needing to get up or soaking through during the night – if you are, this is another red flag. You may find you are using more period products; this could be that you are changing more frequently and the pad/tampon isn't full, but it's fair enough to do 'just in case' changes. If you are soaking thought your products at a rate of knots and changing more frequently because of that, it's a red flag for a heavier flow.

SHADES OF RED

Have you noticed that you have different colours of blood? I know we get a bit squeamish about blood, but it's interesting and is part of the period literacy we can use to help us understand our periods better.

I hear all the time about how gross periods are but, believe me, as an ex-nurse, I can beat you on top trumps of gross things. Periods are, by and large, the least disgusting thing that happens in our bodies – they've just got bad PR. We don't (hopefully) shame kids if they have an accident and wet or poo themselves, which is a natural function of the body. This is the same – blood gets everywhere, and it's amazing we don't leak more often than we do. We have all experienced a nosebleed and how it can look like we have been hit in the face with a bat, and that's probably less than a teaspoon of blood. LEAKING IS A NORMAL PART OF PERIODS, albeit a quite annoying one – the skills we have for getting blood out of things would make us all excellent criminals!

PICK A COLOUR

- **Pink/light red** – This is how a period usually starts and is because it is mixing with cervical fluids, as your period isn't just blood.

- **Brown** – Blood that has had prolonged exposure to oxygen goes brown. If periods start with brown spotting, this is from the previous bleed. Brown blood can also signify a slower flow.
- **Black** – During your heavier days, your blood can be so dark it looks black, and sometimes clots can look black too. The slower your flow, the darker your blood. Sometimes, this can also be to do with the way the uterus sits in the pelvis.
- **Red** – A nice pillar-box red is the optimum colour for a period. It means it's got good flow and is not waiting around in the body for long – this is what a healthy period should look like.

While we don't want the flow to be too slow, we don't want a massively fast-flowing gusher, either! This is moving towards 'flooding' when we are needing to not be far from a loo. The blood of your period shouldn't look thick or very clotted.

A note on clots: small amounts of clotted material is normal, and stringy, blobby bits about the size of your little fingernail are to be expected. These bits and bobs come from your uterine wall. If you are regularly seeing large (50p-size) blobs that resemble liver, this is red-flag material, especially if they're accompanying a heavy flow. Occasionally one might just happen as a one-off – that's fine. What we are always looking for are patterns and regularity, and for changes in all aspects of our period care.

CHAPTER 1 ROUND-UP

- Go through the red flags on page 10 and see if any apply to you.
- Read though the charting section coming up in Part 2 so you can start to understand your symptoms.
- Ask yourself if you have been putting up with period drama and thinking it was OK. If so, what do you need to address?

CHAPTER 2

THE ENDOCRINE SYSTEM: GETTING TO KNOW YOUR HORMONES

The nitrogen in our DNA, the calcium in our teeth,
the iron in our blood, the carbon in our apple pies,
were made in the interiors of collapsing stars.
We are made of star stuff.

Carl Sagan

In a nutshell, the endocrine system is our hormone system. There are over 50 different hormones floating around in our bodies; they are made up of steroids, amino acids and proteins; and each one has a specific role and an associated endocrine gland within the body that secretes it. It is a sophisticated yet delicate system – we blunder about throwing sugar, stress, no sleep, bright lights and more stress at ourselves and then wonder why we feel like we are going to hell in a handcart.

Most of the time the endocrine system just puts up with what we get up to. It computes the disruption we cause it on the outside, twiddles the controls and recalibrates our hormones, and away we go. Sometimes, we have one too many tequila shots and vomit over the bar; it depends how far we try to push things! Our bodies are very good at compensating, but this will only go on for so long – think of the hangovers you didn't get in your 20s compared to the ones you get now. Youth is wasted on the young but, hey, that's hindsight! If we keep pushing our bodies and not looking after them, they start to grumble on the inside, and this then flares up in symptoms, which is how the body communicates to us.

The endocrine system is like a web throughout your body. Hormones get released into the bloodstream and act as chemical messengers. They reach all parts of your body, but only the cells with the correct receptors (like a lock and key) will respond to the hormones.

Hormones act by binding themselves to cells with the appropriate receptors. I think of it like the cheese wheel out of Trivial Pursuit: once the cheese (cell) is full of the coloured wedges (hormones), it becomes that hormone. Hormones need cells to do their work – the cell will carry out the instructions of the hormone because the hormone will alter the cell's proteins or make it build new ones. Hormones need cells to turn specific biological processes in a cell's tissue and organs on and off.

To put it another way, think of the film *Ghost*: hormones are like a ghost Patrick Swayze, and the cells are like a host-body Whoopi Goldberg – the ghost jumps into the host's body and then can physically do things it couldn't do as a ghost.

The health of our cells and their hormone receptors also impacts the response they have to our hormones and their signals. The body uses a miniscule amount of each hormone. Think of chilli peppers: the hottest chilli out there represents our own hormones, and we only need the tip of a cocktail stick to feel its potency. However, synthetic hormones, on the other hand, are like sweet chilli sauce – you need larger portions to achieve the same effects. And the tiniest fluctuations in our bodies have tremendous effect on our physiology.

Hormones regulate by a negative feedback loop (NFL) or a positive feedback loop (PFL). An NFL means if the hormone level is raised, the receptors detect this and tell the gland to reduce the production and amount being released into the body. Conversely, a PFL is where a hormone is released into the body when the body detects it needs it. Childbirth is a good example of this, as the body releases oxytocin to help the uterus contract. The uterus has a lot of receptors for oxytocin and produces more while pregnant – it's as if the body knows what it's doing! The NFL is the more common way for our body to balance things out, as it's easier to stop things to find the balance than to add more in – which is how we do it with medications and is probably why we can feel the side effects.

All of this hormone information is vital because it's all fair and fine to tell people to do or not do something, but if they have no frame of reference as to why they are being asked to notice and perhaps alter a behaviour, it will go in one ear and out the other. If you have an understanding of your body and how hormones communicate, when you come to learn about what can override your natural hormones, I think it helps you turn on the light bulbs and make better choices in an informed way, rather than being told to do something without really knowing why.

When we hear about the importance of exercise, rest, sleep, no light before bed, etc., this is why – because it has an impact at a cellular level in our bodies. We might not think it makes any difference to us because we function doing or not doing those things, but on the inside it is doing something to our cells and hormones and eventually our bodies can't cover up for us any longer, and cracks begin to show.

I do want to mention just one more thing, and that is the relationship between hormones, neurotransmitters and our emotions. Hormones are chemicals found in our blood and neurotransmitters in our nervous system, and they are practically the same – the same but different. This web of cells and their receptors are the hub of communication in the body, and it isn't just the mechanics of the body that change the environment inside, but our emotional state has a big impact too. We are, and have for a very long time, been in a place where the reliance on medication is high – it's seen as the silver bullet to our symptoms. Although medicines have their place, they cannot heal the body in the way that addressing the shit you need to address does.

It might not be the quick way, or even visible at times, but all the work you do to help your mental health – exercise, orgasms, joy, laughter, feeling proud of the wonky scarf you created – actually changes the body's chemistry. This is a side of health that shouldn't be ignored but sadly often is.

THE ENDOCRINE GLANDS AND THEIR HORMONES

The endocrine system works through a bunch of glands scattered in the brain and body. These glands are like signal points to the rest of the body to coordinate your metabolism, energy levels, reproduction, growth and development – so not much at all, really!

The main glands that produce hormones include:

HYPOTHALAMUS
Location: Brain
Job: Homeostasis hub! The hypothalamus takes all the body's information internally and externally over 24 hours and keeps things in balance. It regulates temperature, mood, hunger, thirst, sleep patterns and sexual function to name a few, and it communicates to the pituitary gland by sending signals to each lobe, which then go about sending signals to the rest of the glands in the body.

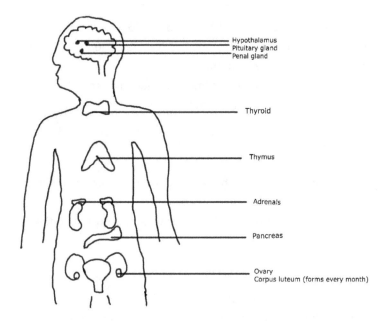

Hypothalamus
Pituitary gland
Penal gland

Thyroid

Thymus

Adrenals

Pancreas

Ovary
Corpus luteum (forms every month)

PITUITARY

Location: Brain – a pea sized glad attached to the hypothalamus

Job: It has two glands, anterior and posterior, together called the master gland (please read that in a voice from a Marvel movie). It gets this grand title because it controls most of the glands in the endocrine system, such as the thyroid, adrenals, ovaries and testicles, as well as producing its own hormones.

Associated Hormones:

Anterior:

- Growth hormone
- Thyroid stimulation hormone (TSH) – activates the release of thyroid hormones
- Adrenocorticotrophic (ACTH) – primary stress hormone

- Luteinising hormone (LH) – see page 26
- Follicle stimulation hormone (FSH) – see page 27
- Prolactin – involved in breast milk production
- Melanocyte hormone – stimulates melatonin to help protect the skin from UV rays

Posterior:

- Oxytocin – contracts the uterus during birth and helps the milk escape during breastfeeding
- Antidiuretic hormone – increases water absorption in the kidneys

THYROID
Location: Front of the neck
Job: The thyroid regulates your metabolism and energy – it's likely that all cells in your body have receptors for thyroid hormones.

Associated hormones:

- Thyroxin (T4)
- Triiodothyronine (T3)

These hormones get down to the nitty gritty of how your body absorbs its nutrients, such as the carb absorption rate in the gut, and also by metabolising fats and proteins, and encouraging the uptake of glucose in your cells, which you need for energy. It is why you can feel absolutely dreadful if your thyroid is out of balance.

PARATHYROID
Location: On the side of the thyroid gland, no larger than a grain of rice
Job: It controls the level of calcium in your body for the cellular well-being of your heart, kidneys, bones and nervous system.

Associated hormone:

- Parathyroid hormone – works with calcitonin, which is produced in the thyroid to help balance the level of calcium in the blood

ADRENALS
Location: In your back, one on top of each kidney
Job: Adrenals control your stress hormones.

Associated hormones:

- Adrenaline and noradrenaline – regulate your fight, flight or freeze response
- Cortisone – part of the glucocorticoid hormones that control your fat, protein and glucose metabolism, which have a key role in supressing inflammatory and immune responses in the body

PINEAL
Location: In the brain behind the eyes, and activated through our eyes as the light floods in
Job: This gland manages day and night cycles, or circadian rhythm, and is light sensitive. It slows in activity in puberty and is generally calcified – becomes hardened – in adulthood, but retains its light-sensing mode.

Associated hormones:

- Melatonin – releases as light fades to help us feel sleepy
- Serotonin – technically a neurotransmitter; your feel-good elixir found throughout the body, particularly in the brain and gut

PANCREAS

Location: Behind the stomach
Job: The pancreas regulates our blood sugar levels.

Associated hormones:

- Insulin – lowers blood sugar, so it isn't like treacle running through your veins
- Glucagon – stimulates your liver to produce glucose and increase blood sugar levels
- Somatostatin – decreases the levels of insulin and glucagon when needed

THYMUS

Location: Behind your sternum
Job: The thymus boosts immunity and is most active during childhood, shrinking as an adult but still having some activity throughout your life.

Associated hormones:

- Thymopoietin and thymosin – aid in the development of T-lymphocytes, which impact your immunity and your immune system

THE GONADS

Ovaries

Location: In the pelvis on the end of the fallopian tubes
Job: They're in charge of ovulation and hormone production.

Associated hormones:

- Oestrogen

- Progesterone
- Testosterone

Testes
Location: Scrotum
Job: Simply put, they make sperm.

Associated hormones:

- Testosterone – affects sperm production, muscle strength and sex drive (in both females and males)

CORPUS LUTEUM
Location: Grown in the ovary in the second half of the menstrual cycle once the egg has been released from the follicle
Job: The corpus luteum produces progesterone and supports a pregnancy until the placenta takes over.

With that, we conclude the whistle-stop tour of the endocrine system!

CHAPTER 2 ROUND-UP

- Your hormones are powerful. You only need a tiny amount to make big changes in your body – having them in balance is key.
- Synthetic hormones aren't going to balance anything. They switch off your own hormones until you stop taking them.
- You grow a new endocrine gland every month, the corpus luteum, provided you have ovulated.
- You are made of many hormones that all speak to each other, so looking after your hormones means taking care of all of them, not just your oestrogen and progesterone!

CHAPTER 3

A DEEP DIVE INTO HORMONES

Hormones get no respect. We think of them as the elusive chemicals that make us a bit moody, but these magical little molecules do so much more.

Susannah Cahalan

So, as you can see, there are loads of hormones, and they are the way our cells – and therefore our bodies – chat to themselves. The reason for the biology lesson is to remind you how our hormones are all connected and that they chat to each other. Also, the next time someone tells you to stop being hormonal, you can say, 'I'm as hormonal as you are, byyyyeeeee.'

MENSTRUAL CYCLE HORMONES

Let's take a closer look at the hormones of your menstrual cycle.

OESTROGEN
There are three types of oestrogen:

- **Oestradiol** is made in your developing follicles in your ovaries and is the primary form of oestrogen during your main period career. It's your 'super sparkly, covered-in-sequins' oestrogen and is potent stuff.
- **Estrone** is made in our gut bacteria, fat tissue and adrenals, and is the oestrogen that we have after our periods have stopped and we are invisible to humanity.
- **Estriol** is the oestrogen you have when you are growing humans.

PROGESTERONE

- **Progesterone is only made through ovulation** – please read that again because it's very important.
- Ovulation is vital for us regardless of wanting to grow humanity because it's how we make progesterone and oestrogen. It is dangerous to have a narrative that suggests it's only important in relation to getting pregnant – it takes away the importance of our bodies just doing their thing.

TESTOSTERONE

- This is made in the ovaries and adrenal glands.
- It helps with growth and bone mass.
- It's also important for all-round general maintenance of reproductive tissue.

LUTEINISING HORMONE (LH)

- LH is produced in the pituitary gland.
- It signals to your ovary to release an egg.
- It determines the length of the luteal phase of your cycle.

FOLLICLE STIMULATION HORMONE (FSH)

- This stimulates a selection of your mature follicles to grow.
- It comes from the pituitary gland.
- The follicular phase of your cycle is marked by the follicles entering their final stage of development.
- During this final stage of development, they start to make progesterone.

Remember: if there's no healthy mature follicle, no progesterone will be produced.

CORPUS LUTEUM

This is the extra endocrine gland that you make every month – how utterly fantastic!

- Its job is to support a pregnancy until the placenta takes over.
- It's reabsorbed back into your body every month if pregnancy doesn't take place.
- You make a whole new one every month.
- It is formed from the follicle that the egg came from during ovulation.
- It dictates the time of your luteal phase because its life span is from 12 to a maximum of 14 days.
- It produces progesterone – without a corpus luteum, we don't get progesterone.

THE HIGHS AND LOWS OF HORMONES

If our hormones are out of balance, they can produce some particular symptoms. This is by no means all of them, but here's a list of the most common hiccups, what happens if your level of a particular hormone is too high or too low.

Oestrogen

Highs: fertility issues (see oestrogen dominance, page 123)
Lows: fertility issues, dry skin, hot flushes, night sweats, tender boobs, irregular periods, mood disruptions

Progesterone

Highs: fertility issues, sore boobs, fatigue, weight gain, mood changes (which probably sounds a lot like the start of a pregnancy, when progesterone is high)
Lows: fertility issues, headaches/migraines, low libido, night sweats, mood changes, irregular periods

Testosterone

Highs: fertility issues, low libido, excess hair, acne, irregular periods
Lows: fertility issues, low libido, weight gain, fatigue, sleep disruptions

Luteinising hormone

Highs: fertility issues, irregular periods, can be seen in PCOS
Lows: low libido, hot flushes, irregular periods, fatigue

Follicle stimulation hormone

Highs: fertility issues, hot flushes, sleep disruption, skin and hair changes, irregular periods
Lows: fertility issues, low libido, irregular periods, fatigue

There are a lot of overlaps – as you can see, too much or too little of a hormone can have the same effects – and it can feel like looking for a needle in a haystack. These symptoms are indicators that hormones are out of balance BUT that isn't the whole picture. All of your hormones dance together, so the reason for the imbalances here might be because of underlying gynae problems, such as endo or PCOS. They could also be out of whack because your stress levels and lifestyle are demanding too much of your stress hormones and these, in turn, are affecting your menstrual hormones. That's why having a whole-body approach to this, which takes into consideration all that is going on with you, proves to be the most effective way of getting to the root cause of any issues.

Identifying hormone imbalances and taking action to re-balance them can help to relieve these symptoms. In the medical model, the approach has always been to medicate and, when that is ineffective, to operate. This has its place at times, but it is often drastic and doesn't take into account any of the other aspects that make up how you can help your hormonal health (such as lifestyle, diet, addressing stress and more). I will be looking at this holistic approach in more detail in Part 2.

Please remember, this isn't a linear process, and your body isn't letting you down and isn't broken – it just needs some TLC. The clients I work with feel lost and hopeless because they feel they haven't been listened to. I have found that even the most ardent hater of their periods can find some compassion for them, once they have vented and someone has said, 'I hear you, and you and your story are valid.'

CAN'T I JUST GET A HORMONE BLOOD TEST?

Of course you can, but there are some things to remember.

• Hormones are always in a state of flux, so getting true readings can be tricky – especially if your period is irregular.

- They are a snapshot of the bigger picture – monitoring and working with your symptoms can be a better indicator of how you are doing in the long-term.
- If you have a longer or shorter cycle, you'll need to take this into account, as most tests are based on you having a 28-day cycle.
- Hormonal blood tests can be costly, and even in countries with public health services, they are generally only reserved for fertility or checking for menopause or have long wait lists.
- There are some great home test kits available if you are happy to pay for them and don't want/are unable to wait.

BLOOD WORK

I'm a fan of getting yearly general blood work done. It is a helpful window into your body and it isn't *that* invasive. When you get bloods done, ALWAYS ask for a printout of the results. You are entitled to this information – they are your test results. I am always keen to look at my clients' blood work. Please don't get fobbed off with 'everything looks fine', it is part of your detective work. The guidelines that are used can be a bit broad within the health service, and sometimes things are missed because of this. Accessing this information in retrospect is much harder, so get into the habit of asking for copies of all your tests.

CHAPTER 3 ROUND-UP

- Read through and familiarise yourself with the symptoms that can be caused by hormonal imbalances.
- Do you show any of these symptoms during your period?
- With the use of charting, can you start to identify any patterns and see where these imbalances may arise?

CHAPTER 4

CHARTING YOUR CYCLE

*Courage doesn't always roar. Sometimes courage
is the little voice at the end of the day that says,
'I will try again tomorrow.'*

Mary Anne Radmacher

If you haven't guessed by now, I'm a big fan of charting your cycle. It's such a powerful way of identifying issues through patterns. Charting is observing the signs and symptoms during your own cycle. You can start by tracking the basics and then adding more elements to your observations as you go, identifying more subtle shifts in your body over time.

Your cycle describes what is happening during the whole month, from one period to the next. It is important to know your cycle length – the time between periods – because this gives you clues to the overall health of your hormones.

To calculate the length of your cycle, start counting on the first full day of your period – this is Day 1 of your cycle. The cycle ends when you start your next period. (If you are spotting but not really bleeding, that is still part of the last cycle.)

A normal cycle can be anywhere between 21 and 35 days, and the 'average' is 28 days – this, however, should not be taken as a gold standard! If you have a cycle that is, say, 26 days on the nose, or is sometimes 25 or 27 days, then that is a normal, happy cycle. If you have numbers that vary widely every month, this is an irregular cycle, and that is not normal. It's also death to all your white underwear.

A regular cycle is important, as it is a signal that your hormones are working as they should. If your periods are varying and you have a cycle pattern that looks something like 26, 30, 22, 28, then your follicular phase and luteal phase will be swinging around all over the place. This is a sign of unbalance; I will be explaining this further in Chapter 6 because, as always, there is nuance with this.

Charting your cycle, and not just your period, is a very illuminating insight into what is going on with your body. Most only chart their periods and miss all the information about their cycles. If you do note the dates of your period, it will be easy to work out your cycle length in retrospect. The day you noted your period is Day 1, and you then count through to the next period – after a few months you will then be able to see if yours is regular or not.

Please note that if you are on synthetic hormones (i.e. taking the pill or having an implant, etc.), you won't be finding anything out about yourself by charting, I'm afraid, because you aren't running the show – the synthetic hormones are.

GETTING TO KNOW YOUR CYCLE

Have you ever wondered why you have felt a particular way, only for your period to arrive and for you to have an 'ah-ha' moment and think, 'Now it all makes sense!' Understanding your cycle is important for many reasons, including keeping an eye on your overall health, tracking where you are in your cycle and having a bit more control to plan things for when you are at your best to tackle them.

I like to use the seasons as an analogy for this because it is something so familiar to us, and it's perhaps easier to remember than the more clinical descriptions. How we feel during our cycle directly correlates with the seasons, too.

You might have thought – like I did when I first started learning about this – that oestrogen and progesterone are the only key players of your cycle. In fact, as we've started to look at already, there are several hormones on the go, and I now want to give you more of an idea about the intricate dance that plays out each month.

Our cycles are seen as something primarily for procreation, and this is indeed a wonderful thing that they do, but our bodies are more than that – we need all these moving parts to work regardless of whether or not a pregnancy happens. I hope, in my work, to shine a light on how damaging that narrative can be, as it can hinder women from receiving the help they need.

Your cycle actually starts in your brain with the hypothalamus, which sends pulses of gonadotropin-releasing hormone (GnRH) to the pituitary gland. This then starts to release follicle stimulation hormone (FSH) and luteinising hormone (LH), which both communicate to your ovaries and follicles.

The following is an overview – your cycle is unique to you and things might not completely align with a 28-day cycle, which is completely OK. Remember: a 'normal' cycle is anywhere from 22–35 days.

SPRING – THE FOLLICULAR PHASE, PRE-OVULATION

The spring part of your cycle is when your hormones are climbing back up again after your period, getting your body ready for ovulation. You might find your energy returning and, just like spring, you are ready to maybe put some brighter clothes on and head back out in the world again. You might find that your clarity comes back – you are feeling more confident and just want to pick back up where you left off before your period. As spring sees life coming back again with all the buds and flowers, so, too, are you.

The reason for this shift is that your oestrogen is on the rise, and this is the action-taker, mover, shaker and fiery hormone. We have several different types of oestrogen (see page 25) but our super-duper one is oestradiol and it is only made in the ovaries. Testosterone is also rising – this is thought to be a male hormone but it isn't, it's produced in all humans. It helps to maintain and build muscle and bone density and boost libido.

FSH is also building at this point in your cycle. It does what is says on the tin – stimulates your follicles to get an egg ready to mature. As it stimulates the follicles, and an egg begins to form, this lead follicle then produces oestrogen. Once the oestrogen has reached its peak, FSH and LH take over once more to nudge the egg over the finish line and help it be released.

SUMMER – OVULATION

This part of your cycle is short and sweet, very much like the summers can be in the UK! However, in terms of your cycle, there is A LOT going on. Ovulation is when your oestrogen and testosterone are at their peak; you most likely feel your most confident, can spin all the plates and feel on top of your game. Very much like summer, you are out and about, the days are longer, you are socialising more, you get more done and the big blue skies lift you up and make life feel that much better.

If you have presentations, talks or anything that requires you to be as sharp as a tack, this is the time to plan them in your diary! Your body is at the peak of its game, so you might as well take advantage of that in other areas of your life! In the summer, you walk with more swagger.

Ovulation seems a bit of a non-event, to be honest, as it only lasts a matter of a day or two, but it really is where it's all at. It's how we make hormones, and if it isn't happening for you, that is a big problem for your whole health. This is where it all comes together, all the hard work your body has been doing to get you here – the dance of the hormones all weaves together and makes ovulation the sensation it is.

AUTUMN – THE LUTEAL PHASE, PRE-MENSTRUATION

When autumn kicks in, the evenings draw darker and, generally, you cling to the notion of the summer – you don't want it to get colder and be indoors, you long for the lazy days of the summer months and want to keep going with that intensity, which just isn't possible. You must harvest and put things away until the next year.

Almost every woman I have worked with hates the autumn part of their cycle. Everything about it is a struggle, and the fight to keep going rather than give into it is where most of us fall down. Put simply, the body just doesn't have the capacity to keep functioning in summer mode during autumn. Summer is for summer, autumn is for autumn – when you think about it, you can't do all the things you did in summer in autumn and vice versa. Winding down in autumn, closely followed by a brief hibernation in winter, allows you to be fully rested, giving you more energy for spring and summer.

I can't stress enough how paring back on the expectation you have for yourself here is paramount. If you are trying to do all that you were capable of with a full tank, why do you think you can do it when it's half-full or nearly empty?!

Immediately after ovulation in the second half of your cycle, FSH, oestrogen and testosterone fall away and LH and progesterone pick up. These are cooler, quieter and more laid-back hormones. As oestrogen peaks, it stimulates the secretion of LH which, together with oestrogen and FSH, makes ovulation happen. LH takes over in the second half; it also instructs the corpus luteum to formulate. The corpus luteum is the ONLY way we make progesterone, so it is very important ovulation happens because it sets off a chain of events that is vital to our health.

As you've read, the corpus luteum is an extra endocrine gland grown every month that supports a pregnancy until the placenta takes over. If there is no pregnancy, it gets reabsorbed back into the body, and a new one will form the following month.

WINTER – MENSTRUATION

This is like being in dark depths of winter, curtains drawn, slouching on the couch watching TV, wanting all the carbs, and feeling like you don't want to talk to another soul. You are inside and don't want to go out into the night again!

Resting is the key to this part of your cycle, as is not demanding too much from yourself. You are bleeding and this is a big deal: it depletes your body, so you need to allow it to 'period in peace' as much as you can. Early nights, delegation and preparing ahead for your needs are ways you can help yourself during this time. We aren't meant to be rollerblading – no matter what the tampon adverts suggest!

The quality of your period will be a culmination of many things: diet, lifestyle, exercise, toxin overload, emotional and physical stress, well-being and everything in between.

I'll repeat this again, because it's important: learning to understand your cycle helps you to understand your body as a whole. Periods that are very painful/heavy are NOT normal and could signify an underlying problem, such as endometriosis or adenomyosis. Absent periods or cycles that go on for 35+ days are also not the norm and could be a sign of PCOS (polycystic ovarian syndrome). These conditions can take a long time to diagnose, partly due to the normalisation of it being OK that periods are a nightmare, and it's always best to get a persistently irregular cycle checked out.

CHARTING YOUR WAY TO SUCCESS

I ask all my clients to chart their cycles. When I ask them if they do, I get a unanimous 'yes', and then I ask a bit more, and it turns out all they mean is they note down the start and end of their periods. All the rest of the money is left on the table.

I know we aren't encouraged or taught to do this, nor have we been given the knowledge to really understand why we should chart – it's just a whole lot of extra fanny admin, isn't it?! All we want to know is it happens, and we are or aren't pregnant – that is really the sum parts of it. It tells us so much more, though. To give you an idea of how useful it can be, studies have started to show that endometriosis can be detected through charting.[1] (Currently, the only way to diagnose this condition is via a laparoscopy, so to say that charting holds a lot of secrets is an understatement.)

I have a free charting course on my website (thewellwomanproject.com), and you can access and download the chart I use. I'm old school, I like pen and paper – it's really satisfying to look back on all of my charts at the end of the year, too. But you can use an app to reach the same results if that's easier for you.

The chart I use is a circle – it has different sections for you to fill in, and you can do it however you like. Some use colour, symbols or stickers – the choice is endless, but I keep it simple by writing the following key pieces of info down:

- The date
- Where I'm at in my cycle (so day 1, 8, 24, for example)
- What I have felt/noticed/experienced that day

Try and do this for every day of your cycle, but don't beat yourself up for missing a day. It might look like this, and you can read this with the *Big Brother* voice in your head too…

- *1/9/22 – Day 1 – Period started, light to medium flow, bright red, no pain, feeling tired, early night for me.*
- *8/9/22 – Day 8 – Feeling energy coming back after my period. CS (cervical secretions) white but dry, no pain, good sleep, libido returning.*
- *24/9/22 – Day 22 – Feeling very tired, need to be in bed early, not so much patience or space for others, feel bloated, spot on my chin, want to eat crumble.*

Charting your cycle will help you to investigate patterns or symptoms that you know you have, but it will also show things that you might not be aware of.

As an example, I get extremely tired a couple of days before my period and could merrily take myself off to bed at 8pm and get a full 12 hours. I hadn't clocked that until I started charting and was wondering why I felt drugged and sluggish at this time in my cycle. Now I make sure I get the right amount of sleep during this time, and that feeling has gone. I also get hungry – like hollow-legs hungry – in Week 3, my autumn phase, and I just want to eat crumble and carbs, all the energy-fuelling foods I can get my hands on. Now I know this, I can prepare for it, make the crumbles ahead of time and enjoy them along with the right sustenance my body requires to have the energy to bleed.

This might not seem like much, but imagine having a stressful task ahead of you and being on your period, or due on. Knowing this and knowing your own personal needs can help you sidestep some of the stress created when you try to push thorough and sack off what you need to function properly.

I leave my chart by my bed, and I fill it in before I go to sleep. It takes less than a minute, and over the course of three months of doing this, you start to build your own personal period toolkit that will enable you to meet your needs, delegate to others and have a bit more control around your cycle and energy requirements.

FERTILITY AWARENESS – WE ALL NEED THIS INFORMATION!

Another way to track your cycle in a bit more detail is through Fertility Awareness (FA). This can and is used very successfully for contraception purposes, or if you just want to be really nosey about your cycle. It is a wonderful way to be in tune with your body and be in the driving seat of your cycle, so to speak. It is a commitment but, when you think about it, you are only fertile for about five days out of every month, whereas guys are fertile ALL the time. I would say it is probably best used in long-term relationships. But it is absolutely worth investigating if you would like to have the autonomy over your body. (I do have a slight grudge that everything about it is about having babies – I couldn't find a thermometer that didn't have something baby related on it! The world won't end because of it, but I find it annoying nonetheless.)

If you are doing this for contraception, I highly recommend you find yourself a teacher and learn this shizzle inside out and back to front. It takes time and practice to be your own expert in reading your charts, and in terms of contraception you want to know you are doing it correctly.

FA tracks three main signs of fertility:

- Basal body temperature
- Cervical secretions
- Cervical position

Let's take a look at these in some more detail.

BASAL BODY TEMPERATURE

You will need a fertility thermometer to check your basal temperature correctly because they give more detailed readings than a regular thermometer. Instead of a reading of 36.5 degrees, it might be 36.56 with a fertility thermometer. You need to take your temperature immediately on waking – before you even get up, check your phone or move about the bed. The reason for this is if you, let's say, get up and go to the loo and then check it when you get back to bed, your temp will have risen, and this can cock up your readings. You want to check your resting temp, so you need to have had at least three hours of uninterrupted sleep to achieve that. Just grab it and stick it under your tongue or arm (under the arm is best practice) and leave it for ten minutes so you get an accurate reading. You would expect to see a rise in temperature around ovulation – this spike signifies that you have ovulated.

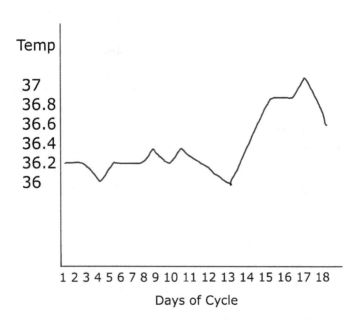

CERVICAL SECRETIONS

Having a look at what goes on in your pants is actually a good habit to get into. Along with the spike in temperature, ovulation creates the snotty, egg white-like fertile secretions. There is an array of things to look for during your cycle in terms of secretions, though, so here is a quick guide to your cervical goings-on at different times in your cycle.

It isn't completely cut and dry – like everything, it depends on other things – BUT starting to notice your cervical secretions is another part of body literacy. Please note: this is isn't icky, it's important and part of your biology, and if anyone tells you otherwise, tell them to sod off.

Period

When you bleed, it isn't just blood that comes out, it's also cervical fluids – not that we really notice because of the red stuff. At this point, both oestrogen and progesterone are usually low. I mean, that's the norm, you might be different because we all are, so that's the beauty of charting – you get to see the real you.

A few days after your period

You still might not notice much in the way of secretions as your oestrogen is still climbing. This is the hormone that gets the cervical juices flowing – as it picks up, so will your secretions.

Moving towards ovulation

As oestrogen picks up, the cervix produces more fluid. At first, it might be thick and sticky or tacky, and then become wetter and creamier, like a lotion. It may look whitish and cloudy, or even yellowish (especially if it's dried on your pants).

Around ovulation

As ovulation is party time, much more cervical fluid is produced. Your vagina will likely start to feel much wetter, and fluid becomes more slippery. Over a couple of days, the fluid becomes more stretchy and clearer. As oestrogen peaks, 1–2 days before ovulation, your cervical fluid can look like a raw egg white or snot that you can stretch between your thumb and finger. Please note that the presence of fertile cervical fluid can't confirm ovulation for sure. Basal body temperature tracking is more reliable for confirming ovulation.

Pre-menstruation

As soon as ovulation is over, vaginal discharge changes and starts to dry up – the amount of fluid decreases quickly. Progesterone is in charge here and tells the cervix to turn the taps off. Secretions may again become sticky or tacky, or just be absent. This leads us back to menstruation, and the cycle begins again.

CERVICAL POSITION

Your cervix is lower and softer during ovulation, and the best way to assess this is to squat down and use a clean middle finger to have a feel. If you do this regularly throughout your cycle (in the shower is a good opportunity), you'll get to recognise the difference.

The three checks (basal body temp, cervical secretions and position) can be used together to track ovulation as a form of contraception. You need to use the information from all three checks together to avoid any risks of a single check producing a false positive and leading to accidents.

If you are just being a bit more curious about your cycle in general, you could just use the temp readings and cervical secretions along with all the other symptoms you are charting to build up the unique picture of yourself and your cycle. I personally like to check my temp and secretions to see if I am ovulating every cycle because I am entering into my perimenopause.

CHAPTER 4 ROUND-UP

- Download the chart so you can get cracking.
- Start getting curious about your period landscape.
- See if you can start making patterns with the symptoms that you find.
- See what your cervical secretions are up to. Can you start to recognise where you are in your cycle from them?
- Can you start to see patterns in your energy levels through the month and where you have more or less depending on where you are in your cycle? Will this help you to plan for your period rather than being taken by surprise?!

CHAPTER 5

UNDERSTANDING PMS

The most revolutionary thing a woman
can do is not explain herself.

Glennon Doyle

Premenstrual syndrome, or PMS, gets its own chapter because it's just so common for us all to feel the emotional fallout of our hormones shifting. I do like Martie Haselton's take on it being called 'premenstrual strategy' instead, because you *can* work with it. Now you have a clearer idea of what is happening in your body, so you can put things in place to help yourself. I want to take a moment here to give a nod to PMDD (premenstrual dysphoric disorder), which is a different kettle of fish entirely. I go into more details about this in Chapter 7. Elements of this chapter will absolutely help, but I want to reiterate that PMDD isn't just bad PMS; it is a severe collection of symptoms that can cause mayhem for two weeks out of every four. As is often the case, research is sparse, but it is debilitating for those that have it.

British doctor Katharina Dalton was the first to coin the term PMS in the 1950s. She studied the link between the collection of symptoms women were presenting and their menstrual cycles. About 75% of menstruating women get some degree of PMS every month. It is a collection of symptoms that generally show up the week or two before our periods. The variety of symptoms is great, as is the intensity of how PMS feels for each person.

When our hormones shift at ovulation from more oestrogen to more progesterone, it's like a power struggle kicks off. We can also feel it with the seasons of the year. When summer starts to dwindle and cool, we longingly look back at the hazy days and wish they were still with us. We can't live in the summer all the time, though – we need balance. Everything in nature has a night and day, life and death, summer and winter. It has to happen because this is how things replenish for the next time around.

WE ARE CIRCLES, NOT LINES

The emotional symptoms of PMS that we have are generally a sign of the things we aren't giving ourselves during our full cycle. If you are trying to push through, and find yourself stuffing all the choc down your face, it's highly likely that you are depleted.

I know it might seem naff to offer another analogy but humour me, I love them! A plant that comes back year after year will flower, die off, maybe lose leaves, but all the energy goes back down to the roots and is stored up for the following summer when it blooms again. During the winter months, you might cover it up to protect it from frost, or feed it with good stuff to allow it to grow strong and make more blooms in its next cycle.

This is exactly the same concept we need to employ for our periods. You cannot be everyone to all people all of the time when you are coming up to your period and while you are bleeding. You simply don't have the capacity for it.

How do I know this? Because my clients tell me, all the time. It is also quite well documented. If you refuse to put your needs first during the window of about 4–5 days leading up to your period and when you actually bleed, you are making life much harder for yourself. I'm an advocate of always putting your needs first, to be honest! You can't pour from an empty jug, as the saying goes. Also, this window might look different for you – identify when your antisocial time is and work with it, instead of fighting it! Think about what might happen if you really leaned into what your body was requesting, instead of ignoring it? Maybe it wouldn't kick off like an angry toddler at you? Just a thought!

There are interesting studies out there that look at the cultural differences relating to PMS and how women around the globe experience it – or not. This, for me, highlights how some of our symptoms are born out of our lifestyles as much as they are our hormones. Toxic productivity and upholding the idea of pushing through regardless of how we feel doesn't work well for anyone. It certainly doesn't work for those with periods.

THE FOUR CHARACTERS OF PMS

PMS can have several different faces. We most likely get a blend of all of them, but let's take a look at these four types so you can get a sense of what chimes with you and what you might do to relieve some of the symptoms. I have labelled them PMS-A, PMS-D, PMS-H and PMS-C.

PMS-A: PMS WITH A SIDE OF ANXIETY
This is the face of PMS that comes with the unwelcome addition of anxiety.

Symptoms:

- Feeling overwhelmed
- A rawness to your emotional resilience, which I liken to having emotional sunburn – your 'skin' is irritated by

feelings of perceived rejection or criticism, making you likely to be more defensive
- Hyper-vigilance, which comes into your surroundings and makes you feel on edge or tense

Why this might happen:

- A hormonal imbalance with oestrogen outshining progesterone
- Adrenal fatigue
- Low levels of serotonin, the happy hormone
- Heavy usage of cortisol, thus activating your fight or flight response

How to help yourself:

- *Sloooow* things right down, mentally and physically!
- Try yoga, meditation, walking in nature or getting more nature in your home.
- Clear things from your diary/schedule that can be moved and prioritise yourself.
- Take Epsom salt baths and/or magnesium supplements.
- Book a massage.
- Try herbs, such as Siberian ginseng and Ashwagandha.
- Get some of my Fuck that Shit potion (see page 150).
- Rest, rest, rest – have earlier nights, sleeping in the dark.
- Create space around you, share your feelings with your family/work friends – if you feel overwhelmed, say so.
- Eat well, eating foods that help to even out your blood sugars.
- Take a look at and address your stress levels in all parts of your cycle.

PMS-D: PMS WITH A SIDE SALAD OF DEPRESSION

Another winner, your PMS can include bouts of depression.

Symptoms:

- Low mood and/or feeling demotivated
- Forgetfulness/brain fog
- Confusion – everything feeling a bit fuzzy
- No energy, like the plug has been pulled out the back of you

Why this might happen:

- Thyroid might be underactive
- Serotonin levels in your boots

How to help yourself:

- Get your thyroid checked via a simple blood test. Your thyroid is your metabolism monitor if you are experiencing fatigue, increased sensitivity to cold, weight gain, joint pain or fertility issues, to name but a few. It's so easy to get it checked and often gets missed.
- Get outside in nature.
- Partake in some activities that are going to give you a boost of energy, such as dancing or taking a brisk walk – something to get the heart rate up.

PMS-H: PMS WITH A TALL GLASS OF WATER

A pretty common one, this type of PMS has some specific physical symptoms around water retention.

Symptoms:

- Feeling bloated, like there's a beach ball around your tummy
- Sore boobs that also seem to have grown
- A bit of weight gain

Why this might happen:

- Having too much oestrogen
- Adrenals may be pumping out cortisol if you're stressed, and also another hormone – aldosterone – which causes water and salt retention

How to help yourself:

- Keep yourself hydrated; this is the time to really hit your two litres a day.
- Eat well – as much as you might have salt cravings here, try not to eat all the crisps.
- Balance your hormones. I suggest Bloody Brilliant Tonic, which is *Vitex agnus castus,* as a herbal support for that (see Chapter 12). Work through this book and tweak other parts of your diet/lifestyle and well-being because that all plays a part too.

PMS-C: PMS WITH A BIG DOLLOP OF EVERYTHING
The one with the cravings face…

Symptoms:

- A desire for all the carbs
- General increase in appetite

- Tiredness and fatigue
- Headaches

Why this might happen:

- Low serotonin – although a sweet treat will only make you feel good for a nanosecond
- Stress and adrenal fatigue, which make you want sugar for energy

How to help yourself:

- Eat well – this is the time to future-friend yourself by having meals prepared and in the freezer.
- Make sure you feel sated after eating or you will create more stress in your body.
- Try to eat so that your insulin isn't poked too much, so opt for slow-release carbs rather than short, sharp sugar bursts.
- Stay hydrated.
- Address your stress levels outside of the PMS arena.
- Rest.
- Do some exercise that slows things down and allows the body space, such as yoga, stretching or Pilates.

SEROTONIN SUPERHEROES

This little neurotransmitter is responsible for making us feel lighter and brighter, and helps keep those anxiety gremlins quiet. It's connected to our hormones because it speaks to them: it has a close relationship with oestrogen, and fluctuations of oestrogen can affect serotonin levels. There are many ways in which you can help your serotonin – firstly, by making sure your hormones are in balance, so working with charting and finding out what your symptoms are and when they crop up. Other aspects include lifestyle, diet, exercise and stress levels.

Herbs that can be helpful include Siberian ginseng – which you will find in my Fuck that Shit blend, which is excellent for anxiety – and also Ashwagandha, which is a fantastic herb known as an adaptogen. This means it really fits in to what it is your body needs and helps support the nervous system as a whole. Feeling low in mood is a common symptom, but not one that we have to put up with.

We can, as I said, have a mix of all four of these types of PMS, as I suspect most of us can attest to. You might well find your PMS changes with each cycle, and looking at these lists can help you see why that might be and show you some tweaks to help you help yourself at this time. We are really just gigantic chemistry sets, after all!

Working with balancing your hormones will absolutely help with PMS, as it isn't just menstrual cycle hormones at play here. This is a full endocrine situation at work, and your PMS isn't really just the 1–2 weeks before your period – it is the whole month. Moreover, it's the whole three months of your follicle maturing. It is your life's work!

CHAPTER 5 ROUND-UP

- Chart your symptoms and see which PMS groups show up for you.
- Take one thing at a time – see how getting more rest or trying a different exercise changes up how you feel.
- Start looking at things from outside your cycle that might be a contributing factor to your PMS too.

CHAPTER 6

UNPACKING RED FLAGS

Growth is painful. Change is painful. But nothing is as painful as staying stuck where you do not belong.

Mandy Hale

Right, I want to unpack my red flags a little further for you because context is everything!

Here is the list again for you so you don't have to keep flicking back and forth. As with everything that is hormonal work, there are a lot of ifs, buts and maybes. I would always rather someone got something checked out rather than thinking, 'Ahh, it's OK, I'm sure this is normal.'

PERIOD RED FLAGS

1. Pain and the use of over-the-counter pain relief – needing to medicate your period 'to get through it' every month, without which you wouldn't be able to function
2. Needing to change your period product every hour or less, and it's soaked and perhaps even leaking
3. Needing to wear several types of period products to go about your daily business because you leak through everything
4. Significant bleeding at night that interrupts your sleep

5. A period that lasts for more than seven days
6. Significant mood disruptions
7. Bleeding outside of your period (sometimes ovulation spotting can happen and that's OK)
8. An offensive odour
9. No period at all and you aren't pregnant
10. Irregular periods
11. Changes to your cycle/period – these might take a while to show and is why I advocate charting your cycle, so you can see these patterns happening before they are worse than they need to be
12. Painful sex – sex should never, ever be painful

Let's take a look at what some of these flags might mean in more detail.

RED FLAG 1 – PERIOD PAIN

Having painful periods is known as dysmenorrhea, and the rhetoric is definitely that it's a normal part of periods – it isn't.

'Pain' is a subjective word and it doesn't really describe things very well. If someone came into A&E with pain, they would be asked for more detail – is it hot, sharp, dull, constant, etc. I appreciate that when I say periods shouldn't be painful, it isn't necessarily that helpful, so let's unpack what that can look like.

Your period will give you some sensations, perhaps a heaviness or mild cramps, because after all, something is happening in your nethers. It shouldn't, however, make you reach for painkillers to get through it. Something is wrong if you need to medicate.

PERIOD PAIN AND PROSTAGLANDINS
Prostaglandins are part of a group of inflammation markers that are made in your immune system and travel to the site

of an injury, illness or infection to aid the healing process. They are released to attend to an acute event in the body, and the inflammation they create causes heat, swelling, pain and sensitivity – this is how the body protects itself. These small actions of inflammation are healthy and normal for the body to experience, but problems can arise when it gets chronic and we have inflammation hanging around the body for a long time.

Chronic inflammation is a state we absolutely don't want our bodies to reside in because it is the root of all disease in the body. When we are showing signs of chronic inflammation, it means that we have more of these inflammation markers floating about our bodies, surplus to requirements. They aren't just attending to acute need; they are cruising about our bodies being meddlesome, like all the best Shakespeare villains. They intercept messages between all the hormones, and this is the precursor of them becoming unbalanced.

Prostaglandins have different roles in the body.

- Some help your blood clot.
- Some thin your blood, which means you can bleed more.
- Some help your cervix to dilate and your uterus contract (to push out a baby or your period).

Although periods are a normal process in our bodies, they are still an inflammatory event and that is why prostaglandins are present. If, however, you are producing too many prostaglandins during your menstrual cycle, it makes sense that you may well experience more pain because there are more of them squeezing your uterus.

Why do we get more prostaglandins?

We get more because our bodies are struggling with inflammation – which is always at the root cause of disease in the body.

Signs of high prostaglandins

We need to look at 'inflammation markers' throughout the rest of the body, as these can be a sign of high prostaglandins. There will be tells of this: generally itchy skin, congestion in the sinuses, coughs, joint pains, digestive upsets, to name but a few. More often than not, we brush these subtle changes aside, but our bodies are telling us they're a bit overloaded. Part 2 will help us look at ways in which we can reduce inflammation in our lives through diet and lifestyle.

RED FLAGS 2, 3, 4 AND 5 – HEAVY BLEEDING

Heavy bleeding is known as menorrhagia (*men-or-rage-e-ah*) and is another normalised symptom. There is some confusion about what should be considered heavy. Some think their periods are unusually heavy and they aren't really, while others have super-soakers but don't think it's an issue – this is why talking about it is important!

We can expect to have some heavier days at the beginning of our periods, but the following are unacceptable symptoms:

- Changing your period protection hourly
- Not being able to be far away from a toilet
- Sometimes being incapacitated by the amount of blood
- Needing to get up in the night to change period protection
- Regularly leaking through period protection during the day and/or night
- Being prone to flooding
- The heavier days of the bleed go on for longer than the couple days that are expected

FLOODING

Flooding is when your flow is heavy and fast and it feels as if your period is literally pouring out of you. It is of concern if you bleed this way for a long time or regularly with every bleed because your iron levels will soon become depleted.

WHY MIGHT THIS HAPPEN?

Conditions like endo, adeno, PCOS and fibroids are *definitely* something to consider if you have heavy bleeding. Some medications can also make periods heavier, so if you have started taking something and notice a change in your flow, bear that in mind.

Higher oestrogen levels are again a culprit for heavy bleeds. If you get one of those stonker bleeds out of the blue, it could also mean that you didn't ovulate that month and had an *anovulatory period* (see page 8), whereby you have a period without ovulating, but your cycle length may well be affected with that too.

The usual suspects of lifestyle, diet and stress can also affect your flow state, so take some time to investigate any changes around these areas of your life too. As we'll see in Part 2, looking after your menstrual health is part of a holistic approach to your overall health that will give you the optimum conditions for your cycle. It's all interconnected.

RED FLAG 6 – MOOD DISRUPTIONS

PMS is considered to be a normal part of the period process and has finally been recognised as an actual 'thing' – for a long time it was considered nonsense! When mood changes get out of hand, however, and you feel that the wheels are beginning to come off, this is a problem. Please refer the previous chapter for more on this, and take a look at Chapters 16 and 17 on the perimenopause and menopause too.

RED FLAG 7 – BLEEDING OUTSIDE OF YOUR PERIOD

Bleeding outside of your period means seeing blood when you wouldn't expect to. This isn't getting your period a few days earlier or later. This is seeing bleeding mid-cycle and is something to get checked out. Occasionally, spotting can happen, but if it's prolonged or happening frequently, please go see your doctor. Also, if you have gone through the menopause and you are bleeding, see your doctor immediately.

Spotting is very light bleeding that can occur either side of your period, outside of your normal period; sometimes it can appear at ovulation. You may have experienced it after a smear, for example. You might only notice it on the loo paper. If it happens, the most you would need to wear, if anything, is a panty liner. Spotting in expected circumstances is nothing to worry about; it's just a red flag when it turns up and it's out of your norms.

WHY DOES SPOTTING HAPPEN?

There are many different reasons that spotting can occur, so it is something to keep an eye on. Again, it's about being aware of what is 'normal' or usual for you, and paying attention if things change. And if you are concerned about it in any way at all, get yourself checked out. Spotting might be caused by any of the following:

- Using any type of synthetic hormones – these can cause breakthrough bleeding due to the changes in hormones in your body
- Fibroids – fibrous tissue in the wall of the uterus
- Polyps – small cysts that can grow on the cervix
- PCOS
- STIs – especially chlamydia
- An infection of the uterus or cervix
- Perimenopause
- Uterine cancer – a red flag for this is noticing spotting once you're through the menopause

As well as spotting, if you have any pelvic pain, fevers, changes in frequency and length of bleed, or you shouldn't be bleeding anymore, see your doctor.

RED FLAG 8 – AN OFFENSIVE ODOUR

Thrush, or candida, is a common yeast infection. We usually know we have it due to an insanely itchy labia/entrance to the vagina. You might notice a thick, white, cottage cheese-like discharge that has a slightly yeasty smell to it. Getting the occasional bout of this happens, and isn't cause for concern. However, if you are getting infections regularly, say, 3–6 infections a year, I would treat that as a red flag. It could indicate a more widespread issue with thrush throughout your body.

Bacterial vaginosis (BV) is something we can get if we clean our vulvas and vaginas too much. Normally, it shows itself with a watery, greyish discharge that smells like fish. Vulvas might well become itchy, which makes for a bit of a vicious circle with wanting to clean them more, etc. Your vagina is self-cleaning – you don't need any of the products you find in the feminine aisle.

Soap goes on the outside of your vulva only, and clean water goes on the inside, and that's it. BV might happen once or twice in your lifetime and, again, having regular or frequent infections like this signals that something in your immune system might be off-kilter.

I have worked with many clients with both of these complaints, using herbal products with great success. Usually people come to me because the conventional medications have stopped working effectively, as our bodies can become resistant to them when used regularly – more on that later.

RED FLAG 9 – NO PERIOD AND YOU AREN'T PREGNANT

Anovulatory cycles can be part of the perimenopause (see page 215) and can also be caused by other specific conditions. Please refer to the next chapter for more information on this, especially concerning PCOS (polycystic ovary syndrome).

RED FLAG 10 – IRREGULAR PERIODS

'Menstruation' comes from the Latin words for 'moon' and 'month'; the term 'period' also has Latin roots meaning 'recurring cycle'. So, your period is meant to come at roughly the same time each month, every 21–35 days, give or take a day or two.

When a cycle starts to swing about and it's 22 days one month, 34 the next, then back to 25, or it's more than 3–4 days different every month, you have a cycle that is irregular. You may well have always had a cycle like this, but that doesn't make it right, and there will be an underlying cause for it.

The big question here with irregular periods is if ovulation is occurring, as anovulatory periods can be irregular. Without ovulation there is no progesterone made.

Early and late periods that fall before 21 days or after 35 days are a type of irregular period. Both of these can happen because of anovulatory cycle, illness, stress, dieting or the peri. If you have a long cycle, then you have had an extended follicular phase. If you have a shorter cycle, then the follicular or the luteal phase will have been shorter. Sometimes these can happen with no harm done, but it is absolutely worth keeping an eye on.

That's because, in some cases, it can be because we have a specific condition such as endo, adeno or – highly likely – PCOS. It can usually be seen during the beginning of our period careers and perimenopause, but this is what we would expect to see. When you are in your period career, however, an irregular period can be a sign of imbalanced hormones, not just oestrogen or progesterone, but also thyroid. It can affect fertility and is basically fanny admin Russian-roulette style.

RED FLAG 11 –
CHANGES TO YOUR CYCLE/PERIOD

Any changes to your cycle should make you prick up your ears, but you will only notice this if you are recording it. Changes might take a while to show, and this is why I advocate so strongly that you chart your cycle, so you can see these patterns happening before they are worse than they need to be. Otherwise, we tend to only take notice of the blindingly obvious symptoms! Again, cycle changes could be down to perimenopause, or they could be a specific condition revealing itself. It could also be your body reacting to stress, diet or lifestyle factors. Charting is invaluable to help us find the clues in our cycles. Take a look at Chapter 4 to find out more.

RED FLAG 12 – PAINFUL SEX

Sex shouldn't be painful, but there are times that it could be the case, due to:

- Dryness of the vagina
- Prolapse
- Vaginismus
- Pelvic floor issues

If you are in your perimenopause or menopause, the lower oestrogen levels that come with them can affect how much natural lubrication that you make. This can cause vaginal dryness, which can make sex uncomfortable at best, and excruciating at worst. Using lubrication isn't just for when you get to the peri or menopause, however. There is no shame in needing to use it. Vaginal dryness is generally linked to lower oestrogen levels, and these can fluctuate not only around peri/menopause, but also when breastfeeding, post-ovary removal (oophorectomy) or because of immune disorders. Also, things like smoking, douching and some medications can affect the lubrication of the vagina.

I was hearing about dry vaginas a lot from my clients, so I came up with a natural moisturiser/lube called Love your Labia lip balm. It has been a total hit and led to a lot of happy flaps. Its natural ingredients of marigold and lavender make it perfect for such a delicate area of the body, and all lips deserve a lip balm! You can find it on my website, thewellwomanproject.com.

VAGINISMUS
Vaginismus is a condition whereby the muscles of the pelvic floor and vagina involuntarily go into spasm and become very tight, often making pelvic exams, inserting tampons and penetrative sex impossible. It can happen as a teen or develop later in life.

Seeing a pelvic floor physio is helpful. Dilators are used to help those that have vaginismus to work with their bodies. With time and patience, this is a condition that can be overcome, and normal service can resume.

Sex is something that ties in with our nervous system. It is something that is vulnerable to us, and if we are too in our heads, then the chances of those barriers being able to come down are heavily impeded. This can make for sex that perhaps feels uncomfortable or numb, and it's a case of getting out of our heads and into our bodies. Some of us just take more warming up to let loose, and that is absolutely fine. Allowing yourself the space to explore that with a partner or solo is a gift to yourself, as is savouring pleasure rather than rushing it and getting it off the to-do list. No wholesome orgasms were made this way.

THE PELVIC FLOOR

The pelvic floor is the name for the hammock-like muscles that keep all your bits where they should be, married up with other tendons and muscles. They all form the base for not just your uterus, but your bladder and bowel too. I'm currently working mine out and I suggest you do too, every day. It is a great bit of self-care to look after these muscles as much as you would any other. They can be put through their paces if we have humans, but they're also susceptible to our hormone changes during puberty, pregnancy and menopause.

Prolapse

If this doesn't make you get going with your pelvic floor homework, I don't know what will. There are four types of prolapse you can have: uterine, bladder, bowel and vaginal. You can also have more than one at the same time – sorry about that.

A vaginal prolapse is when the vagina slips out of place. The other three are when those areas of the body drop down into the vagina. There are varying degrees of prolapse, and sometimes the organs can be felt and seen out of the vagina. Needless to say, it's uncomfortable; you can feel a dragging, heavy feeling in your tummy, vagina and lower back; and obviously, sometimes, you have visible proof too. When our pelvic floor isn't as strong as it needs to be, it can't support the weight of the organs above it. The potential causes of a weak pelvic floor have been explored in the pelvic floor section. Prolapse can be reversed naturally, but you will need the right support team for that. My best piece of advice is don't sit on it – if you think it could be happening to you, get on it. It's much easier to fix a mild case than one in later stages.

CHAPTER 6 ROUND-UP

My sincere hope is that no red flags are being raised, but I know that won't be true for everyone. My takeaways for you in from this section are:

- Chart, chart and chart some more! You want to be a nerd about your own body. Writing things down is solid evidence for you and whoever you work with.
- Trust your gut and the symptoms you are presenting with. Remember: the normalisation of a lot of rubbish symptoms are deeply ingrained.
- Don't be fobbed off. If you don't get the answers and services you require, get a second opinion and ask all the questions. Sadly, this is a bit exhausting and time-consuming, but you are worth that effort!
- Work with one thing at a time so you are clear in your approach, rather than trying to scattergun because that makes things difficult to pinpoint.

CHAPTER 7

SPECIFIC CONDITIONS

The truth will set you free, but first it will piss you off.

Gloria Steinem

Chronic gynae conditions are sadly more common than we think. The stats make for sober reading, but the real travesty is the amount of time it takes to get a diagnosis. It can and does take years for formal diagnoses to be made. The damaging narrative that it is, for example, normal for us to experience painful and heavy bleeding, is largely to blame.

It's a sad state of affairs that so many are suffering needlessly, creating the perfect storm for the whole body to unravel mentally, emotionally and physically. Since the pandemic, wait times have increased across health services, and women's health has taken an extra hit. Some are looking at waiting over a year just to get the ball rolling. Approximately 80% of women waiting for gynaecological care found that their mental health has declined because of the waiting times – and pain has been cited as a significant factor in that.[2] This goes to show how women's health care has been deprioritised and needs an overhaul.

I have helped so many of my clients to reach a diagnosis of the conditions in this chapter by simply listening to them and helping them put the pieces of the puzzle together. In general, 23% of women and people with gynae organs feel they aren't listened to when seeking help from health professionals for gynaecological care.[3] This only aggravates the problem of trying to find the right support and answers. Although it isn't the best news in the world to find out you have a health problem, it is crucial to know as then you can really start to give your body what it needs.

The bottom line with the conditions I'm talking about in this section is that no one really knows why we get them. There will be answers to that; we just haven't found them yet. My personal belief is that it is a mixed bag of everything we look at in this book.

I know I felt a terrific sense of relief to find out I had endo and adeno. I was starting to think maybe I was losing my mind – being constantly told everything was OK, when I knew instinctively it wasn't. My whole period career suddenly fell into place, and I could see the timeline of events so clearly.

ENDOMETRIOSIS (ENDO)

This condition is defined by tissue that resembles the endometrium (uterus lining) forming on the *outside* of the uterus. Endo hasn't been classified as an autoimmune disease (a condition in which the body's immune system attacks itself, creating inflammation), but it does have the hallmarks of an autoimmune disease (characterised by widespread inflammation in the body), and it has the capacity to create autoimmune responses in the body. There can also be a genetic link to this condition in the matriarchal line of the family.

Symptoms are wide and varying but common ones include pain, heavy bleeding, painful sex, abdominal bloating, ovarian cysts, lightning bum (shooting pains that feel like electric shocks up your bum), fatigue, pain when opening the bowels, urine frequency, fertility issues and pain outside of your period.

Endo is a full-body disease, which means it can and has been detected in the brain, lungs and bowel, as well as in the uterus and pelvic cavity. It causes adhesions within the pelvis (although adhesions can be found in other parts of the body). These adhesions are like sticky cobwebs that can fuse parts of the body together, and this causes pain. The endo tissue found in the pelvis and body, in effect, has a period with your period, so bleeding can be seen in the places where the tissue is present.

The severity of endo has a grading system going from 1 (less severe) up to 5 (a clusterfuck). This doesn't always correlate with the levels of symptoms experienced by the person, though. Someone could have Grade 5 endo and not have pain, and a Grade 1 could be rolling on the floor. So, really, I use the grading system to tell me the amount of endo present and then talk to the person who has it to glean the rest of the info.

Oestrogen dominance is something that is associated with endo. Suffice to say the relationship with endo and oestrogen is complicated. It does seem that endo sufferers have symptoms that show oestrogen is higher, but it's not as simple as to say that's the direct cause. A retroverted uterus (a uterus that sort of folds back on itself, thereby not allowing a good flow with your period) is also a possible contributing factor – again, not backed up by science, but everyone with endo I have ever worked with has had one, so go figure!

Shockingly, one in ten women have it and take, on average, eight years to get a diagnosis. Also, it is a myth that having a baby, taking synthetic hormones or getting a hysterectomy will cure it. Currently, a laparoscopy is the definitive diagnostic tool, although patients are sometimes offered ultrasound, CT and MRI scans; even though these can miss the disease, they are far less invasive. I do wonder if a laparoscopy is the 'gold standard' approach, or if we have doctors that don't always know what they are looking for. I know there are experts in this field that have diagnosed patients via vaginal exam. It still seems quite hit and miss, and the patient can carry a lot of the burden of seeking the best care. I work with the symptoms, which are a constant guiding light. When people come to my door, they are usually feeling more than a little desperate and hacked off with the system, but I do see my clients' symptoms dissipate with the use of herbs, lifestyle changes, body work and diet changes. These remedies are tailored to their personal requirements and problems that they arrive with. Going forward, they are then armed with the skills and knowledge to help maintain the balance they seek.

ADENOMYOSIS (ADENO)

This is a disease about which very little is known, and it can sometimes accompany endo. Adeno is a characterised by the thickening of the uterus wall, which is termed 'soggy' or 'lumpy' uterus by health professionals – nice! The endometrium grows into the uterus muscle, making it appear lumpy and thick on an ultrasound scan, which is how it can be diagnosed. It can take a while to get a formal diagnosis because adeno can be masked by endo, or doctors fail to look for it.

It is very similar to endo in that it has links with higher oestrogen signs and symptoms. It's difficult to know how many people have it or how long it takes to be diagnosed because there has been very little research into the condition. Again, its cause is unknown, but I would surmise it will be an autoimmune situation, a lot like endo is.

All I know is that when sufferers become aware of their symptoms and start tweaking things as part of a holistic approach to their bodies and lives, symptoms can start to abate, and they achieve some semblance of a better quality of life.

Symptoms, again, can be a long list, but the most common ones are pain in the abdomen and pelvis, heavy bleeds, large clots, an enlarged uterus, painful sex and fertility issues.

Ablation is sometimes offered – where they laser off some of the lining of your uterus to reduce the bleeding – as is a hysterectomy, which would get rid of adeno altogether, as it is contained within the uterus. Synthetic hormones can be offered to help mitigate the symptoms, but this it isn't a cure.

POLYCYSTIC OVARY SYNDROME (PCOS)

PCOS is a metabolic and hormonal disorder with multiple and complex symptoms affecting many hormones in the body. Usually, those with PCOS have more androgens (hormones seen in higher levels in males) than those without it, and their ovulation can be affected – sometimes going missing in action for months at a time – which reduces progesterone. Insulin and cortisol performance can also be erratic.

Some of the more common symptoms include:

- Irregular ovulation
- Acne
- Weight gain that is stubborn to shift
- Polycystic ovaries
- Fertility issues
- Insulin resistance/insulin imbalance
- Irregular periods
- Thyroid imbalance
- Cortisol imbalance
- Hair loss from head
- Excess body/facial hair
- Pelvic pain
- Chronic inflammation in the body

To unpack a couple of these further, insulin resistance is when the body becomes less efficient at dealing with glucose in the bloodstream. If left untreated it can then develop into type 2 diabetes. Insulin resistance is a very common symptom in more than half of those that have PCOS. Sometimes connected to this, PCOS sufferers can also make too much cortisol, which can increase the risk of thyroid and insulin problems, and bring along the emotional side of the cortisol stress hormones flying through your body. Finally, PCOS can affect the thyroid, making it overactive or underactive. As a general rule, if it's overactive, you will be more meerkat, and if it's underactive, more sloth. So, you see, lots of vicious circles and chicken-and-egg conundrums going on as well!

PCOS is another condition that is very common – with one in ten women having it – but takes a long time to diagnose. It can be overlooked because each symptom is often looked at in isolation, rather than as the collection it really is. It is a multi-layered condition that is tricky to navigate. There is no known reason why some people suffer with PCOS, but genetics are thought to play a part.

POLYCYSTIC OVARIES (PCO)

Having polycystic ovaries, or PCO, is not the same as PCOS and is not a disease. It's the diagnosis given to those who have ovaries that have multiple partially mature follicles that look like lots of cysts. Not everyone who has PCOS has PCO on their ovaries. Not everyone who has PCO has PCOS. This is why it's important to look at the symptoms being displayed in your body.

OVARIAN CYSTS

Ovarian cysts can come in a smorgasbord of options – you can get them because you have an underlying condition that predisposes you to them, or they could appear just for the hell of it. You might know you have one, you might not; they can come and go. They also have a risk of twisting and bursting if they get large, which is something none of us wants to happen.

There are different types of ovarian cysts:

1. **Functional cysts** – These are when a normal process in the body goes a bit off track and a cyst forms.
2. **Follicular cysts** – These occur when the follicle that the egg would normally pop out of doesn't pop out an egg, but carries on growing into a cyst.
3. **Corpus luteum cysts** – These happen when the follicle the egg came from turns into the corpus luteum, and the opening where the egg pops out gets blocked, thus creating a cyst in the corpus luteum.

We most likely never know about these things happening because they are usually symptom-free – although if you are hot on reading your body, you might notice it. They usually clear up on their own after a few cycles.

There are other cysts that might occur and hang around. There are many but the two I want to mention are these:

1. **Dermoid cysts** – These little mutant orbs are made up of hair, teeth, skin and other random body parts – a right little shop of horrors! They aren't connected to hormonal shifts per se, and they are the most common type of cyst. They can grow to large proportions. Interestingly, they are thought to be there from birth! They are only troublesome if they get too big for their britches and start creating problems.

2. **Endometrioma/chocolate cyst** – These are reserved only for the chosen many that have endo. They sound like they're not so bad but get their common name because they are filled with blood. They are a symptom of endo.

The symptoms are similar for both:

- Discomfort in your lower back and thighs
- Nausea
- Fainting
- Bloating/swelling in your belly
- Painful sex
- Pelvic pain before your period
- Pain when going for a poo
- Sudden onset of pain out of the blue that makes you sweat, feel faint, is relentless and is usually in the pelvis/side of body (front or back) – **if you get this, go and seek medical assistance immediately**

The main issue for cysts is if they get so large they start pulling and twisting on the ovary they are attached to, or if they rupture and burst their debris into your pelvic space. I don't know about you, but I don't want the little shop of horrors running amok inside my body, nor do I want the internal equivalent of a spilled hot chocolate!

Cysts can be felt through an internal examination if they are big, and imaging (such as ultrasound, CT or MRI) can also show these. Surgery through a laparoscopy may well be required if they are causing problems in there; otherwise, it's a case of keeping an eye on them. I have helped lots of clients to significantly reduce a cyst's size or reverse it over time.

One final piece of advice on this is to go and have an osteopath appointment if you have had a large cyst removed because your body will be wonky when it's not there. It will help you to no end to be back in alignment.

FIBROIDS

These are benign growths that can grow in and on your uterus. Sometimes they can get big – even make you look a bit preggos – and surgery might well be needed to remove them if that is the case. They generally vary from teeny tiny to hefty hugies and anything in between. There might be just a singleton or a gaggle, and you may not know you have them at all.

Symptoms can include:

- Heavier bleeds
- Pain in your pelvis lower back and legs
- Bulky, bloated tummy that doesn't go away
- Constipation
- Not emptying your bladder fully
- A frequent need to wee

Sometimes fibroids don't cause too much bother and can be left to their own devices, and they can shrink during the menopause. Treating them by balancing hormones and tweaking lifestyles and diets can also go a long way in improving life with them.

PREMENSTRUAL DYSPHORIC DISORDER (PMDD)

PMDD isn't just 'bad PMS'. It's likened to having a total Jekyll-and-Hyde moment during your cycle. Funnily enough, why it happens has not yet been identified. However, I'm of the persuasion that it's caused by an imbalance of hormones, or a body that is very sensitive to any change in hormones. Looking at all the other facets of a person's life is very important with this, too. Although it can include the same general symptoms as PMS, PMDD can last much longer as it kicks off in your luteal phase. It could last a few days or could be the whole blimin' time – ugh. It starts to build a dread in those that have it, as they worry for themselves and those around them as they slip off into the abyss every month. And it understandably becomes pretty all-consuming, either being in it or worrying about being in it.

PMDD can look like:

- *Extreme* mood changes, irritability, anger, sadness, hopelessness, anxiety, lack of energy or interest in things you enjoy. You may find it hard to concentrate, feel overwhelmed, out of control or very tense, maybe lashing out at those around you or feeling like you are being rejected.
- In some cases, this can lead to suicidal thoughts which, sadly in some cases, have been acted upon.
- People liken it to self-destructing, having an Incredible Hulk moment and then having to do damage control once it has ebbed away again. The cycle is exhausting.
- It can strain your relationships, social life, work and family life. There isn't anything that doesn't get involved with the fury this can create.

The usual care offered for PMDD is synthetic hormones and antidepressants, but there are other routes if these don't suit you. Herbal remedies can be really helpful, and I have had great success working with clients to balance out their hormones and get their diet and lifestyle needs in check. It is also important to address any emotional and psychological stuff going on. Our hormones are so sensitive to our outside world and environment. If you are dealing with trauma, be it with a little or big T, seek help to resolve it.

PELVIC INFLAMMATORY DISEASE (PID)

This is an important public service announcement because PID can really fall under the radar. PID is a bacterial infection of the uterus. It can, and often does, go undetected for too long. It's often caused by a sexually transmitted infection but can also be triggered by our own bacteria found in the vagina, and it isn't something only young women get. It can lead to fertility problems and creates pain – we've got enough of this going on already without inviting another unwanted house guest! The two main STIs that cause PID are chlamydia and gonorrhoea.

Symptoms might include:

- Pelvic pain
- High temperature
- Foul-smelling vaginal discharge
- Painful sex
- Pain when passing urine
- Irregular periods

This is a bacterial infection so it will need to be treated with antibiotics. The damage it can cause can be irreversible, and antibiotics won't fix that damage. Get the sexual low-down from your partner and use protection in the form of condoms. Get checked and then swing from the chandeliers to your heart's content! Also, douching isn't advised, as it washes away your good bacteria. Remember that your vagina is self-cleaning, so we don't need to be poking about in there or doing a deep clean. Nothing but clean, fresh water should be used on your inner labia – certainly no soap needs to be inside you.

If you have the urge to clean something thoroughly, take it out on your home, car or handbag. Don't succumb to media and the patriarchy telling us we have to smell like a bouquet of roses down there. We need to smell of vulvas, that's it.

CHAPTER 7 ROUND-UP

- Track your symptoms.
- Research these conditions more to see if they resonate with your experiences.
- Take your findings to your healthcare provider for further investigation.
- Read the rest of this book to see where you can bring in some changes yourself.
- Don't suffer in silence. If you need to talk through something, reach out and ask for it. I am always at the end of an email.

CHAPTER 8

BEING SEEN AND HEARD

*My mission in life is not merely to survive, but to thrive;
and to do so with some passion, some compassion,
some humour, and some style.*

Maya Angelou

There is a lot of talk about how women aren't listened to properly in the medical system, and every single client I have seen can attest to this. I have even experienced this myself, and I worked in the system for years! I don't want to bash the health service, as it gets enough of that politically, and there are wonderful individual practitioners out there who are striving to do their absolute best. However, the studies speak for themselves. Women are fed up with being told nothing is wrong, having pain minimised and being made to feel that they are a nuisance.

Professor Brené Brown talks about how medicine is one of the most shame-based educations. Patients, particularly female patients, are made to feel foolish or ashamed – either deliberately or subconsciously – on so many occasions, and it is very damaging. This culture of shame starts at med school, ramps up during residencies and carries on all the way through careers. It crosses specialties, is rampant everywhere, and is absolute currency in some specialties.

No one can work in this amount of toxic soup and not be affected by it. The legacy of hysteria still lingers to this day and persists mainly through a drastic lack of education and by living in a society that has a male-centric lens on health.

THE MEDICAL PATRIARCHY

This started way back in Ancient Egypt and Greece. The Egyptians believed that females had a womb that wandered about their body, causing no end of trouble.[4] As for the Greeks, renowned scientist and philosopher Aristotle hypothesised that 'the female was "a mutilated male" whose development had stopped because the coldness of the mother's womb overcame the heat of the father's semen.' On top of that, it was thought for thousands of years that a woman was a poorly made man – their genitalia was the same as a man's, just turned inside out. Physician and philosopher Galen wrote, 'Just as mankind is the most perfect of all animals, so within mankind, the man is more perfect than the woman, and the reason for this perfection is his excess heat, for heat is Nature's primary instrument.'[5] Although this belief was finally dismissed, its legacy can still be felt.

'I've got a bad toe, Barbara.'

'It's your uterus, Margaret. Go shake it back where it belongs. And remember to smile while you do it.'

Women's hormones have always been looked at as something of a sickness in medicine. We have been subjected to so many barbaric practices and procedures over the years, all in the name of curing us from our bodies.

The word 'hysteria' comes from the Greek for womb, as it was seen as a purely female complaint. The Victorians inadvertently invented the vibrator, believing that orgasms helped release the hysteria. (This is hilarious given how prudish they were.) And the American textbook for psychiatric diseases only removed hysteria from its list in 1980!

The legacy of this patriarchal approach to medicine is seen, sadly, in massive gaps in data and research. Even today, medical textbooks, posters and models predominantly use male bodies or skeletons to reflect what they are talking about. For example, clitori have been excluded from textbooks, the female anatomy is often added as a side note in books if it's significant to a particular health topic, and learning about the menopause has only recently been added to medical curricula.

Furthermore, nearly all studies for medications are done on men or male animals, the implication being that it is too costly, too complicated and subject to too many variables to use women. We aren't a smaller version of males. Women's bodies are very different, from how we metabolise food to our immune systems, right down to the makeup of our cells.

One study that did get funding looked at the impact of endometriosis on a man's sex life.[6] Another was proposed to study whether women with endometriosis were better looking than those without – there was such uproar about this one that it didn't get approval. However, it made it through by changing the title to: 'Does having more oestrogen in your body keep you looking younger?' Interesting, perhaps, but in the cold light of day, there isn't enough research being done on curing diseases in women's health.[7] I think studies like these can wait.

Patriarchy in medicine can lead to insipid views and the oversimplifying of women's health issues, which can lead to gross oversights. Patriarchy can be upheld by women (through internalised misogyny), and there is a belief that women can be more sympathetic to fellow women, but that isn't always the case.

We cannot ignore the stats that show how women are dismissed more readily than their male counterparts when it comes to health. And women of colour have a greater chance of being overlooked, as if it's not enough to have a bias against your sex alone! Some dangerous beliefs perpetuate in medicine, such as the idea that black women are able to tolerate more pain, leading them to not always getting the pain relief they need.

As of 2024, all medical students will have to complete training on all women's health matters, as part of the UK government's first-ever women's health strategy scheme. I think this is fantastic, but I do want to ask the question, why wasn't it deemed necessary to learn about women's health before then?

GASLIGHTING IN MEDICINE

Gaslighting is a term used to describe a form of psychological abuse whereby a person or group makes you question your reality. It leaves you feeling anxious, confused and with an inability to trust yourself and your version of events. It's not easy to pinpoint, but it feels icky, like something has washed over you.

Gaslighting can happen in all forms of relationships, but in a healthcare setting and especially around women's health, gaslighting affects outcomes. It is very powerful to understand medical gaslighting because it helps you to build the advocacy for your own health. It's the difference between being able to choose what you want off the menu and the waiting staff telling you what you are having, regardless of your dietary requirements.

Gaslighting in medicine might look like:

- **Countering** – 'Are you sure about this? Are you sure this really happened?'
- **Withholding** – Refusing to engage in conversation, for example, not telling you everything that has gone on and

simply saying that everything is OK or your results are fine, even when you ask for them specifically – this is a common one!

- **Trivialising** – Belittling or disregarding your feelings or experiences
- **Denial** – Pretending to forget events or how they occurred
- **Diverting** – Derailing a conversation to change its focus
- **Stereotyping** – The person may intentionally use negative stereotypes about a person's gender, race, ethnicity, sexuality, nationality or age to manipulate them, making them out to be irrational or over-sensitive – this is a big one!

Medical gaslighting also occurs when the medical professional dismisses or trivialises a person's health concerns based on the assumption they are making it up, exaggerating, or that it is all in their head.

A study in 2009 found that doctors were twice as likely to attribute coronary heart disease symptoms found in middle-aged women to mental health conditions than they were when middle-aged men presented the same symptoms.[8]

Women are more likely to die from complications if they have had surgery performed by a male surgeon than they are if their doctor is a female. What makes this really icky is that it isn't the same the other way around – there is no difference in outcomes if a woman operates on a man versus a man operating on a man.[9]

Women are less likely than men to be believed when they are in pain, according to a study in 2021. The pain gap, as it is referred to, shows that women are more likely to suffer from chronic pain conditions and yet less likely to get pain relief than men. Women are more likely to be told to try psychotherapy,[10] or sent away with sedatives[11] or anti-anxiety medication.[12] I'm gonna stick my neck out here and say this has got strong hysteria vibes! Sometimes it doesn't feel like we have moved further on! These internalised beliefs hamper the speed of diagnosis for all disease, but especially those centred around our hormones and periods because so many already carry the belief that it's OK for them to hurt in the first place.

The rhetoric that women are hysterical, emotional and sensitive beings still runs very deep when it comes to our overall health, but never more so than in relation to our uteruses. They are seen as something through which we can be controlled – we have basically been operating under one helluva propaganda movement for literally hundreds of years.

BEING YOUR OWN KICK-ASS ADVOCATE

It's important for us all to play our part in countering gaslighting in medicine. I encourage you to be assertive when dealing with the medical system and to advocate for yourself and other people whenever you can.

Remember, it's OK to do any of the following:

- Ask your doctor for copies of any tests you have had – blood tests, x-rays, ultrasounds, scans. All of these are yours, and I recommend you always ask for a copy of them.
- Ask to see your notes. Sometimes you might have to pay for them, but whether it's notes from the doctor or a hospital, you are allowed to look through them.
- Ask if you can get a second opinion if you don't feel you have been heard, or if you just want one for peace of mind.
- If you are needing to see a doctor for a specific condition, it's OK to make sure that the person you see is an expert in that condition. It's OK to ask them about their knowledge in this particular field – gynae doctors might know about fannies but they might not know a whole load about ones with endo or PCOS. Seek out the experts who deal with that all the time.

- If you are needing to have surgery for your endo, for example, it is imperative that you have excision over ablation, as this makes a MASSIVE difference to your outcomes. An ablation doesn't get rid of it like excision does. It's the difference between getting the root out of a weed growing in your patio compared to just chopping off the leaves – if the root is still there, it will grow back.
- It's also OK to talk with your surgeon about what they plan to do and to disagree with those plans – for example, my surgeon wanted to remove my ovary, and I asked her to save it.
- You don't have to take medication you don't want to take, if you don't feel it's right for you. To clarify, if you need it to stay alive, take it, but if you don't and you want to explore other routes and your doctor can't advise on that, it's OK to decline or say you want some time to think about it.
- Have your questions written down ahead of time or, better still, take someone in with you and have them prepped for what you want to ask. You may also want to record the consultation so that you can listen back to it.
- Please always complain if something is wrong – change will never happen if complaints aren't made. I know that we are so vulnerable at these times, but it is so important people complain about things. I used to help people fill these forms out when I was a nurse, as I'm a huge advocate for getting your voice heard.
- Ask for things to be explained to you again or in more detail if you don't understand them. Ask about the medications and how they work. Ask about any research you have found. And keep asking until you feel happy with what you are doing.

The reason advocating is hard is because you are in your experience, and you are feeling, existing and coping with less-than-desirable symptoms. You get scared, think you are going mad – especially when you keep getting told there is nothing wrong. And you are TIRED, so damn tired, banging your head against a desk repeating, 'I think there is something wrong with me,' only to be told there isn't, or go have a baby, or that periods are meant to be this way, so take the painkillers and have a nice life.

When you are on the receiving end of information about your health, you get tunnel vision – you hear probably about 30% of what is said to you because your brain goes into overdrive about how it must be something bad and you are going to die. It's very normal to think like this – your brain is smart *and* a drama queen all at the same time. Because of this, you often can't stay rational, take on the information being said and ask the questions you need to ask, all at the same time. This is why taking someone with you that has the questions you want to ask but can also recall the consultation is really helpful.

Advocating for yourself has never been so important. Telling your health professional your expectations and desires is a very important aspect of care, and their ego shouldn't come into it – they should work alongside you rather than saying, 'It's my way or the highway.' The health professionals that have a better working approach with their patients make all the difference.

POSITIVE SELF-TALK

I invite you to take a moment here to think about how you talk about yourself and express things to others about your hormones and periods. Are you bashing yourself with the concepts that have been handed down to us? Are you empowering your sisters, daughters and friends to challenge the narrative that they are being ridiculous? Switching up the way you talk to yourself and others about your hormones and periods can be a real game-changer. It's OK to be a bit off when you are having your period, but say that. 'I have my period right now and I'm not feeling on top of my game.' This is vastly different to saying, 'I'm a hormonal wreck, sorry, I'm being emotional.' You might feel a wreck or emotional, but I really implore you to not give away your power by using language that was gifted to us by men who thought we were mutilated males – just a thought!

I quite like saying, 'I'm having a power surge,' or 'I'm on my period, I may be very truthful,' or 'I'm feeling tired because my body is losing blood' – this one shuts people up pretty quickly! Feel free to be as graphic as you like; the mention of clots earns you full house points. Make a game out of it: *how many points will you give yourself for the words you have to say?* This can be pretty hilarious. Don't get mad, get mischievous. We don't have to love our periods, but we can work with what we have, and making things funny is always helpful. If I can make a whole audience make a barf noise, I feel very proud of myself!

STORIES

I reached out to my community, and here are some of the negative experiences they have had in the medical world. This might be a painful read, but these are real, honest stories, and they are important to share. Some sound quite unbelievable, which just goes to show the far-reaching effects felt by careless or misogynistic medical talk. As you'll see, sadly, some of these interactions were with female doctors, perhaps showing the level of internalised misogyny and other prejudices still around in society, and how far we still have to go.

'It's just part of having periods.' That's what the doctor told me when I used to have to be in bed for two days every month because I was in so much pain. – *Katie*

A doctor told me, 'Are you thinking of having a baby soon? For most ladies, things settle down after having a baby.' – *Lauren*

When I was having one of my post-kidney-donation check-ups, I saw a female doctor I hadn't seen before, and she asked about how it had been managing my recovery whilst looking after my children. I told her I didn't have any children and was child-free by choice. She replied that was a shame and a waste, as I was clearly a very loving maternal person, implying that the fact I'd donated a kidney made me an ideal mother. – *Sadie*

I was always told my symptoms were weight-related, and that stung more than being told my severe pelvic pain was basically all in my head. I told my doctor to go back to medical school and that my pain wasn't psychosomatic. Years later, after being fobbed off repeatedly, I kicked right off, and they found extensive endomitosis and bowel adhesions with ovarian cysts attached to my bowel. – *Jules*

After having twins, I diagnosed myself with diastasis recti, as no one had done a post-natal check on me. I got my belly grabbed and shaken by the female doctor, who told me my issue was that I was fat and I had to lose weight, rather than looking for anything medically wrong. I left the doctors and cried all the way home that day. Twelve years on, I still have it, and I'm so scared to go back to the GP to discuss it. Instead, I try to heal it with Pilates. – *Vicki*

I had just had an emergency episiotomy, both my newborn son and I were in complete shock, and I was trying to breastfeed for the first time. At this point, the surgeon knowingly smiled at my then-partner, leant across my post-birthing body and said, 'Don't worry, I've put an extra stitch in to make sure it's nice and tight.' That fucking stitch caused me so much pulling and pain that I took painkillers for the first six months of motherhood while sometimes crying because the scar tissue was tugging. – *Allison*

I asked to be sterilised after my second baby as I had had a mini stroke. I was told no, because if something happened to one of my kids, I'd need to have another. I did have a third baby that I was advised to terminate due to the risk to my health. I then had another mini stroke and was told that I should have listened to my GP and ended my pregnancy. I put a complaint in as they should have listened to my request to be sterilised. I obviously wouldn't be without my child now, but this was almost 14 years ago. The system is still so broken, and it's scary as a mum to three girls – I'm having to teach them to stand up for their rights, question everything and not take 'no' for an answer where their health is concerned. – *Lindsay*

CHAPTER 8 ROUND-UP

I hope that reading through this chapter and these experiences shows the need for self-advocacy. It is your body and your experience, and you deserve to be seen and heard with the utmost care and dignity.

Getting a second opinion is always a sound idea – we use sounding boards many times a day about all sorts of things in our lives. This is no different. If your gut says, 'Hmmm, I'm not 100% sure about this,' then get someone else to check it out. Peace of mind is important.

When you go for an appointment, take someone with you or record it. As patients, we don't take in very much information because we are worried. Someone else that is removed from the situation can help you make sense of it. You can have them ask pre-set questions, request further clarification, etc.

Get copies of your blood work and test results when you are with the doctor, as they're so much harder to get in retrospect. I always advocate that you get printouts of everything for your own record. If you change doctors or work with someone like myself, then we have all the information.

Above all else, be kind to yourself. I hear a lot of hate speech given to bodies about how stupid they are or how they've failed, etc. That really doesn't help the cause, and I know it's not ideal having illness and problems, but beating yourself up over them isn't going to help one iota. If you can't bring yourself to be loving, that's OK, but be neutral. Seriously, no hate to yourself.

CHAPTER 9

A QUICK HISTORY OF SYNTHETIC HORMONES

To bring about change, you must not be afraid to take the first step.

Rosa Parks

I will be honest with you here: I took the pill for ten years and, for the most part, I thought it was great – because I didn't know any better. I didn't have informed choice; it was just what everyone did. I'm telling you this because I don't want you to think I'm sitting in some lofty position of never having used it and judging the shit out of anyone that has or does. Since stepping into the world of women's health, I have gained a greater understanding of synthetic hormones, and it has stopped me from taking them ever again.

The first experiments in making synthetic hormones came in the 1940s. Progesterone was extracted from wild yams and synthesised, but at the time there wasn't funding to go any further with it. It wasn't until the 1960s that synthetic hormones hit the market big time.

During the testing phase in the '50s, the women involved were convinced they were pregnant because all their periods stopped. No amount of reassurance would make them think otherwise, so the pharmaceutical company listened and added in a breakthrough, or withdrawal, bleed. This is a break in taking the hormones, usually 7 days in a 28-day cycle, and the drop in hormone levels in the body makes the lining of the uterus shed. This pretend period is there to make you think your body is working as it should be, that taking these hormones hasn't altered your period in any way.

Millions of women now use some form of synthetic hormone, be it the pill, patch, implant or rings, and more than 50% use it for more than just birth control – it is widely used to deal with problematic hormones.[13] It has become the go-to medicine offered.

In this chapter we'll take a look at what this means for your body. Note: I use the term 'synthetic hormones' to encompass all forms of hormonal contraception – oral, injection, implant, coil (IUD) and rings.

PRETEND PERIODS

The period you have while taking synthetic hormones isn't a true bleed. It is a forced bleed due to the mix of hormones you are taking, and it doesn't provide any insight about your own period or cycle, which could happen every 5 days, every 28, every 60, or not at all. The 'pretend period' is just there to make you feel like nothing has changed.

While you are taking synthetic hormones, you have no natural cycle, and your hormones are switched off. You are taking hormones that override your own, turn them off and make you sterile for the time you are on them. This is why, when you stop taking them, it can take up to a year for your own fertility and cycle to get back into the swing of things.

Since the synthetic hormones turn your hormones off, they can't really balance anything out. Once you stop taking them again, you will be right back where you were before you started.

WHAT SYNTHETIC HORMONES DO TO YOUR BODY

Taking synthetic hormones affects every cell in your body, and can cause changes to your:

- Brain
- Digestion
- Energy
- Weight
- Mental health

You are not in charge of your body while you are on them, and the frightening thing is that so many of us can and do spend our whole lives on them. Perhaps you take a little break to have children, if you choose, and then go back on the pill, and then on HRT, and you are on hormones for life. It's quite a sobering thought to think you are being medicated from, potentially, the age of 16 until you shuffle off this mortal coil.

There is no other medication that a well person would take for this long. We are only fertile for approximately five days each month, yet we are the ones turning off our fertility by medicating for years and putting up with some pretty awful side effects.

POSSIBLE SIDE EFFECTS OF SYNTHETIC HORMONES:

- Reduced libido
- Weight gain
- Mood changes
- Depression
- Sore boobs
- Spotting

- Breakthrough bleeding
- Headaches/migraines

The complaint I hear most often from my clients is that they are put on the synthetic hormones, and they might start out OK, but then their body kicks back and symptoms arise. Or, it is a shitshow from the beginning.

BALANCING OUR HORMONES

When you take medication, it can't discern the needs of your particular body – it just does what it was made for. So, if you take the pill because your moods are feral, for example, the synthetic hormones in the pill will affect the good feelings as well as the bad. You can't cherry pick; it works as a blanket, and it covers everything.

The pill was never intended for the use that is has now – it was for short-acting spurts. It now has become less about stopping pregnancies and more about curing period problems, which it doesn't do, it just band-aids them. As soon as you stop taking it, all the symptoms that were there will come back again. And sometimes symptoms will return even while taking the synthetic hormones, or they never stop in the first place.

I work with a lot of women who have come off hormones. Generally, they stop for a specific reason, but then find they feel completely different off them. They realise that a fog has cleared, they feel different, and that they really don't want to go back onto the pills, patches or implants.

During your period career, your body changes, your cycle changes, and how you metabolise synthetic hormones will also change. This is why some things work for a bit and then they don't. The longevity of good health comes from fixing the underlying cause, or at least knowing what the underlying cause is, so you can apply some logic to how you want to proceed with a treatment plan.

Just being given synthetic hormones arbitrarily, without even getting to the bottom of why someone has painful or heavy periods, could well be masking an underlying condition such as endo, for example. This just stalls that person getting the right and proper care. Synthetic hormones DO NOT cure any menstrual issues – they might well give some relief, but getting to the root cause should be the goal, not just papering over cracks.

WHEN SYNTHETIC HORMONES SHOULD BE USED

In some circumstances, such an early menopause or a full hysterectomy, where ovaries are removed at a young age, taking synthetic hormones is really important so that your body has the hormones it needs to sustain itself. Early menopause or a full hysterectomy before the menopause are situations that require support because they sit outside the norm of what your body should be doing. It's also a massive shock to your body to have hormones one minute and none the next if you have a full hysterectomy. This is when hormones are beneficial because they are supporting a system that isn't working or has been taken away. When the menopause occurs at the right stage of life, it happens gradually and, more importantly, it is meant to happen then. It isn't a requirement to take hormones during this time, but they are an option. See Chapter 18 for more on this. If you are in a position whereby you are unable to make your own hormones, or have them taken away suddenly, this can be detrimental to overall health, and replacements are, on balance, beneficial.

WHEN SYNTHETIC HORMONES CAN'T BE USED

It's worth noting that some women can't take synthetic hormones due to specific conditions or a medical history that make them unsuitable. Then what? I always say that you have so much more control over your hormones than you think. In terms of working with your body to help hormonal imbalances, the whole of Part 2 of this book is going to be looking at the ways our diets, lifestyles and moving our butts can help.

USING SYNTHETIC HORMONES FOR CONTRACEPTION

We have sex recreationally far more than we do to procreate. A lot of young women choose to use synthetic hormones because they don't want to get pregnant as they start to explore their sexuality. I find this very hard as a feminist – I think every woman should have the right to choose what is right for her; however, I don't think we are getting all the facts when it comes to synthetic hormones and our health.

Yes, access to contraception should always be there, but I think we should also be encouraging women to learn body literacy. To understand our bodies, we need to sow seeds from a young age. I'm so tired of the dogma that if you teach young people about sex, it turns them into sex-crazed delinquents! What it actually does is encourage young people to ask better questions and understand consent and the workings of their bodies, rather than gleaning most of their information from magazines and porn sites.

In the Netherlands, age-appropriate sex education begins in primary school and continues until students graduate.[14] The Netherlands has one of the lowest teen pregnancy rates in the WORLD.[15] I think that speaks for itself, doesn't it? We might not want to think about our kids having sex any more than they want to think about their parents doing it, but don't we owe it to them to help them make better choices, to go out in the world armed with knowledge about themselves?

They might not use all of this knowledge now, but it might resonate later in life, so nothing about it is wasted. Ultimately, it doesn't matter when you start learning about yourself, it all counts. All I ask is you don't just blindly follow the path that has been set out, the one that is born out of oppression, control and distrust of women and their bodies – you deserve way better than that.

If you would like to avoid using synthetic hormones as contraception, the following options can be a good fit:

- Condoms
- Withdrawal method
- Fertility charting – taking temps/monitoring cervical secretions/feeling for changes to your cervix
- Copper IUD

It isn't for me to say one way or another what you do with your freedom of choice. I myself feel conflicted because it is so very complex. I have used synthetic hormones without knowing any of this information, and now I do I think I would have thought twice about it. What I will emphasise is that you should do your homework in detail, and this book is a good starter for that. If you are taking synthetic hormones, some of the elements of this book won't work because your hormones are effectively switched off while you are taking them. Working on nutrition, lifestyle, stress and exercise, though, is never wasted. My hope is that you gain knowledge from this book, and you are able to perhaps address the problems for which you are taking hormones in the first place. Most women now are on hormones for hormonal issues rather than contraception – but they don't fix your hormones, they're a band-aid. We deserve more than to be medicated for potentially our entire lives. I don't know of any other drug we would take for life that has the potential to do us harm and changes how our bodies work at such a cellular level.

It's a tough conversation to be had, mainly because I feel it isn't one that happens a lot of the time; usually, we are prescribed something that we really know little about. There is no judgement from me. I am so passionate about women's health and there being freedom and choice, but that also needs to come with balanced information so you can make informed choices. Taking control of your own health is a radical act of self-care, you are your own best advocate, and empowered, educated women further empower and educate women.

CHAPTER 9 ROUND-UP

- Does the information here change anything for you? How does it land? There are no right or wrong answers, but how they make you feel is important. Please take some time to explore these questions.
- Do your homework. Read more about synthetic hormones, ask the questions and look at research until you are satisfied with your own choices.
- If you are taking synthetic hormones for issues you have with your periods and hormones, would you like to come off them and try another route? No right or wrong answers here, either!
- If you are on them and you are happy and it's working, great. You have to do you; all I ask is you go in with your eyes open. But remember: there are always other options – nothing in life is a one-size glove for everyone.

PART 1 ROUND-UP

In Part 1, we have set the groundwork – a better understanding of our bodies, our hormones and how the pieces of the puzzle fit together. It's as complex as it is simple, a lot like magic, which is how it can feel when things start slotting into place. I never get tired of the smiles and shocks that happen when someone's hormones get straightened out and their life gets back on track. It's the best feeling and best result for all concerned.

Moving on to the next part of the book, we will zoom out and take the wider view, looking at a whole-body approach to supporting menstrual and period health. I know that the notion that a period doesn't have to hurt is more than a bit alien to us all, but I can't stress enough what an important piece of information that is, because believing the alternative stops us from getting the care we deserve and need.

PART 2

WHAT YOU CAN DO ABOUT IT

You must love and care for yourself because that's when the best comes out.

Tina Turner

In this part of the book, we will unpack the other facets of hormonal health care and take a look at external and internal factors that have an impact on our hormones and periods.

The body is like a large department store, and the linear view would have us stay on the ground floor poking about at the hormones in the pelvis department. However, a lot of the time, we need to get the escalators up to the other floors to see what is going on there. We want to be bringing our menstrual hormones all sweetly in flow and get all of the elements of the endocrine system working well with each other.

Part 2 is also about taking some personal responsibility for our hormonal health. It's all too easy to blame things we can't see, i.e. our hormones, when we might actually be contributing to the problem ourselves by not making the best diet and lifestyle choices, or maybe being stress-heads and not addressing that.

We are going to be taking a holistic view and looking at the things we need to be the best version of ourselves. It can be uncomfortable peeking in the dark corners of ourselves. It can also seem a bit left-field to go there, but it's where a lot of the juicy stuff resides. I'd say 95% of the work I do with my clients is unpacking the upper floors of the department store, before we drop back down to the ground floor and zone in on period health.

Also – and I will shout this from the rooftops till the cows come home – putting yourself first isn't selfish, it's how you get stuff done. Perhaps you've never had practice at setting boundaries, saying no, or sitting in the slightly uncomfortable place that is putting your needs first. Trust me when I say that it gets easier with practice!

Right, let's dive in...

CHAPTER 10

NUTRITION

Our food should be our medicine, and our medicine should be our food.

Hippocrates

Nutrition is everything to our health – we are what we eat. Our food has a direct impact on our health, sometimes immediate, sometimes gradual. In terms of menstrual health, what and how we eat can have a great impact, which is great because it means that we can tweak our diets and see results in our health.

Every one of us is different, and our bodies need different things. None of us are getting out of this alive. Some health coaches can be dogmatic, suggesting we live only on mung beans soaked in the sweat of unicorns. If the advice isn't followed, then you will get sick, and it will be all your fault. I don't believe this attitude is helpful – no one is motivated by being shamed and blamed. My belief is if you give people the information, they can make educated choices that serve them best. I work with my clients to help them figure out what will work best for *them*, not what I think they should do.

There is a balance with everything, and I'm all about the 80/20 rule: 80% sticking with the things that make us feel our best, and 20% face-planting into the cake. My clients get this drummed into them because food is to be enjoyed. I don't want a life without cake. I just don't eat it all that often so, when I do, I really fucking enjoy it.

There are times we flip this 80/20 ratio and face-plant into cake a lot more often – life may throw a curve ball of magnificent proportions, and we just have to get through it as best we can. Nothing is permanent, and I remind my clients all the time that the 'falling off the wagon' in any area is important. It generally shows you how well things were working for you beforehand and is a reminder of how far you have come.

I believe that as long as you strike a balance of doing what is best for you and allowing yourself some wiggle room, your body will be able to cope with most things. Also, bear in mind that all the fear about whether or not something is good for us perpetuates the stress we are looking to avoid.

This is ongoing learning, so what worked for us in our 20s is different to our needs in our 30s, 40s, 50s and beyond. Looking to work *with* the changes in our bodies, rather than fight them, is a big advantage, however difficult this can be in a society that values youth while poo-pooing ageing, wisdom, wrinkles and experience.

FLAMING INFLAMATION

In this chapter we are going to be looking at some food groups that can exacerbate inflammation, which can make periods worse and upset our hormones. As with everything to do with hormones, there is nuance; sadly, I can't tell you to just stop eating cake and everything will be OK. It's the processes that certain foods kick-start in your body that are the key to nutrition. There is so much to it – I could fill a book just on this subject! These chain reactions that occur with the following food groups have a significant impact on our hormonal health.

They imbalance our hormones, hinder detoxification and interact with other hormones and systems in our body. Nutritional changes can and do have an impact on every facet of period health like PMS, pain, flow and energy. Having good nutrition is vital for your whole period career, from when you start right through to the peri, menopause and beyond.

'Wholefood' is just that – food that has minimal or no processing. This is without doubt the best food to eat. Home cooking is also preferable to ready-made food because you know what goes in it. I realise that I'm in a privileged place here. I have the capacity to cook every day and afford the best ingredients I can. So, before we head off on this exploration, I urge you to come to this section with an open heart. Do the best you can, and make small changes that escalate into big changes. Slowly weeding out things from your diet is also better than trying to do everything at once, which is impossible and overwhelming.

Reading the back of packets can be a very helpful way to educate yourself on what's in your food. If I can't pronounce an ingredient, I generally assume it isn't something I really want to be eating anyways! Items at the top of a product's ingredient list are present in larger proportions than items lower down. For example, cereals can be a surprising source of sugar – cornflakes don't taste particularly sweet, but sugar is their second ingredient. If we dump a load of sugar on our cornflakes and then have sweetened milk, you might as well start your day with pic'n'mix and be done with it!

As you read this chapter, start to make notes on what foods you think make you feel less than OK. Start to look through your cupboards and look at the ingredients for yourself. I think it is way more powerful to do this than have me tell you. There is a lot of crap that goes into food we are unaware of – opening our eyes to it is the first part of the process. I liken our efforts to eat the best we can to the horse-meat scandal. There is nothing wrong with eating horse per se, but I want to know I'm doing it.

There are five major food groups that contribute to creating inflammation in your body:

- Sugar
- Alcohol
- Wheat/gluten
- Dairy
- Vegetable oils – rapeseed, corn, sunflower, etc.

Understanding what these groups do in and to our bodies is hugely eye-opening. All this can feel a bit doomy, so at the end of the chapter, we will look at the foods that help our periods, and I have offered alternatives to things where I can. Let's start with everyone's favourite bogeyman – sugar.

THE SWEET STUFF

There are three types of carbs: starch and fibre (complex carbs) and sugar (refined or simple carbs). Sugar isn't just the white stuff – it also derives from refined carbohydrates like white rice, pasta, bread and white potatoes. Everything we eat is a carbohydrate; they aren't to be feared, just understood.

Complex carbs aren't complex to find, fortunately; they get their name because of how they are molecularly structured. Ideally, we want a diet higher in complex carbs than refined ones. What happens when we eat refined carbs is that they affect our insulin, which interacts with all our other hormones – remember, they are all connected and communicating.

Our bodies need glucose (sugar) to survive – it gives us the energy for every conscious and subconscious task – and this is why we need to eat regularly. We don't need to add it to our diets, though, because our bodies make glucose from the complex carbs, proteins and fats we eat.

It's not just the spike and crash of insulin that is the problem with a diet high in sugar and refined carbs; it also affects how our hormones work. The irony is we crave sugar for an energy boost, but it ends up making us feel more lethargic. Reducing our sugar and refined-carb intake really does increase our energy levels because our insulin stabilises.

If you are craving sugar around your period, then have a look back at Chapter 5 and see if there is anything that can be addressed there, because munching on all the cake can make PMS symptoms worse.

When we eat a meal that is high in sugar and/or refined carbs, the spike in insulin affects a specific protein that helps bind excess oestrogen and testosterone, which is then excreted from the body via the liver. If we are low in this protein because of eating a diet high in sugar and refined carbs, then we have more oestrogen floating about our bodies, which causes imbalances, and we see symptoms like PMS, hot flushes, pain and fatigue, to name a few. Insulin also increases the production of testosterone; this then converts into even more oestrogen and is stored in our belly fat.

Diets heavy in sugar make huge demands on our insulin, and it starts to lose sensitivity; this is known as insulin resistance. I will talk more on this later, but it is a key player in hormonal health.

I invite you to do a sugar and refined carb audit for a week; the amount consumed can be pretty surprising. It's easy enough to do: keep a food diary and then look up the sugars that are contained in the foods you have eaten. It's recommended we eat no more than 30g a day. You can do this type of audit for any food group you are looking to investigate in your diet.

SWEETENERS – A WARNING

Sweeteners – for example, aspartame – are best avoided like the plague; they are the work of the devil. Sugar-free products tend to use sweeteners that are carcinogenic.

Aspartame also damages your gut bacteria. A much better sugar substitute would be stevia, which comes from the leaves of the stevia plant. In fact, I've grown stevia before, and it's the most bizarre experience to bite into a leaf that tastes like a spoonful of sugar!

What does sugar do?

As we know, a steady blood sugar level stops hangry outbursts and helps stabilise the hormones. It also allows the liver to do its job filtering out all the extra junk in our bodies. An excess amount of sugar does a couple of things to us. Firstly, it can create insulin resistance in the body, which can be a precursor to Type 2 diabetes.

Insulin resistance occurs when the cells in our bodies don't respond to the insulin we make. The cells can't mop up the excess glucose in the bloodstream efficiently, so we pump out more insulin. This makes our blood sugar levels look like a mountain range. Of all the things we want to be linear in life, blood sugar should be at the top of the list.

Secondly, sugar clogs up our cells, which gives the immune system the hump and triggers it to send out the inflammation markers, a process that increases overall inflammation in the body. As we discussed in Part 1, inflammation should be a short-lived response to an immediate problem. If we are constantly filling our bodies with things that create inflammation, we are increasing our chances of unbalancing our hormones throughout the endocrine system and therefore creating the perfect storm for period and hormonal issues to arise.

Where does it hide?

Sugar is found in some pretty obvious places, such as soft drinks, tonic waters, sweets, chocolate bars, cakes, desserts, pastries, breakfast cereals, flavoured yogurts, biscuits, dates, honey, agave, coconut sugar and fruit juices. But it also hides in a huge number of everyday products, so be aware of the following on your food labels:

- Sucrose
- Fructose
- Molasses
- Maltose
- Glucose
- Dextrose
- Syrups – glucose, fructose, maple and corn
- Honey
- Treacle
- Coconut sugar
- Rice syrup
- Date syrups

Refined carbs have no fibre or nutrients in them and affect insulin in much the same way as eating neat sugar. Some examples of refined carbs include:

- White bread
- White pasta
- White potatoes
- Pizza dough
- Pastries
- Breakfast cereals
- Baked confectionaries

When you check the ingredients of anything you eat, the higher up the list that any of these sugars appear, the larger the quantity of them the food contains. Also check how many types of sugar are on the list, sometimes consecutively. Natural sugars are still sugars – they aren't healthier because they come from a coconut instead of a sugar cane.

To tell if a food is high in sugar, check the packaging where it gives the amount per 100g/ml. High-sugar foods contain more than 22g per 100g, and low-sugar foods contain 5g or less per 100g.

Kicking sugar completely is pretty impossible, but lowering it and eating more complex carbs that slowly increase your insulin, rather than creating massive spikes, is a winner. We will explore this next.

SUGAR SWAP

If you are looking to reduce your sugar, here are some hacks you can try:

1. **Increase your complex carbs.** These are foods that are whole and have retained all their fibre, such as brown bread, wholewheat pasta, veg, fruits, sweet potatoes, quinoa, beans, pulses and lentils. Also, adding in more protein and healthy fats will give more sustenance than the refined carbs, which rocket through your body.

2. **Start your day on the right foot.** If you are consuming a sugary breakfast – cereals or toast and jams – you are setting yourself up for a crash. Try starting your day with eggs, porridge and fruit, homemade granola or a breakfast buddha bowl. Having more protein and longer-acting carbs will maintain a more even blood sugar. If you find you crash through the floor mid-morning, just tweaking your breakfast can be a game changer.

---

3. **Find sweet alternatives.** Although still sweet-like, 'toffee dates' are an amazing alternative for a sugar hit. I like to slice the date and remove the stone, then add a blob of peanut butter and a chunk of raw cacao, and I have myself a Snickers bar! Even though dates are high in fructose, they have fibre and other nutrients.

Fruit is also always a winner, eaten whole or mixed in a fruit salad. I even make ice cream out of banana. Slice two bananas into discs and put them in the freezer. Remove them when they are frozen (a couple of hours later) and bung them in a food processor. Whizz them up until they are thick and blended, and they taste like ice cream! I enjoy mine with a blob of nut butter – yum!

Another hack for balancing your blood sugar levels is to have your sweet treat with a meal. That way, your body digests it all together, rather than having a standalone sugar hit. Ideally, you don't want to be snacking loads, but eating at regular meal times. If you aren't sustained by what you're eating and getting *hangry*, then you probably need to re-examine your diet.

Please remember: the aim isn't to be perfect, the aim is to be curious and explore what it is your body needs. When you eat food you like, your body is going to react – it's biology, none of us can help that. Understanding this helps you to choose better for yourself, and that affords you a lot more agency with your hormones.

BOOZY BOOZERTON

In my work, I often find that bringing up the subject of cutting down on booze meets more resistance than sugar! Alcohol vandalises your gut bacteria – that's why it's used in hand sanitiser, after all. Your liver has to work harder to detox, and alcohol also drains your glutathione protein – an immune-balancing antioxidant which helps rid your body of excess inflammation. This means if you have more oestrogen floating about your body, your liver can have a harder time frog-marching it out of your body. Remember: oestrogen can bind to receptors through food and external environmental toxins, so having a liver that is working effectively helps to purge the body of the stuff that doesn't serve us.

I knocked booze on the head about three years ago now. My intention was to give up just for a bit, and here I am. I didn't drink loads, but generally necked more than the recommended allowance. I just woke up one morning having had a couple of glasses of wine and felt like poo, and I knew it wasn't serving my body. So, I stopped. And I was really shocked to see how much my skin, body shape and general puffiness (that I didn't even know I had) improved. I was also surprised at how I had to look at things head-on because I didn't have a glass of wine to dull the senses – that was unexpected!

Booze is also often served with sugary mixers – we all remember the days of Archers and lemonade or Malibu and Coke, right? No wonder we all needed cheesy chips at 2am to regulate that sugar crash – thank goodness we also danced our shimmery asses off as well, because that exercise would have helped, too... and we were in our 20s, let's be fair.

The NHS recommends we drink '**no more than 14 units of alcohol a week, spread across three days or more**. That's around six medium (175ml) glasses of wine, or six pints of 4% beer. There's no completely safe level of drinking, but sticking within these guidelines lowers your risk of harming your health.'[16]

If you are having trouble with wild hormones, I would suggest you try cutting back your alcohol intake or stop drinking it altogether for a while and see what happens. The world won't end, I promise, but your feral hormones might.

BOOZE SWAP

The non-alcoholic beverage situation has come a long way in recent years. Personally, I prefer the low-alcohol version of beer (<0.5%) rather than the alcohol-free (0%), as the 0% can taste very sweet. These can be an easy swap. There are some amazing 0% gin, rum and vodka spirits that make lush cocktails or a G&T. The wines and fake fizz are still a bit hit-or-miss and can be quite sweet, but the industry is listening, which means it will keep evolving and getting better.

This might sound daft, but get yourself a fancy-pants glass to drink your beverages out of. Add in all the mint and lime you want to your soda water. Some bitters are also great for adding a bit of bite. Make your non-alcoholic drink a bit special and feel smug about how much better it is for you, with a bonus point for no hangovers too.

GLOOPY GLUTEN AND WEARY WHEAT

If you get symptoms from eating wheat and/or gluten, then you need to listen to your body because it's telling you that it doesn't like it.

This is one of the food groups that some folks with cast-iron insides can eat with no issues at all. Some will have some sensitivity to it and therefore will swerve it, but won't explode if they accidently eat some; and then there are the handful that can't take it at all.

The reason I touch on wheat and gluten is that people can be intolerant to it, and that is important to know. The reasons for this can be varied: you may have had an intolerance since childhood, developed it later in life, or it could be to do with a condition you have, like endo, for example.

Allergies and intolerances aren't the same thing; sometimes we can grow out of an allergy and then be able to tolerate a small amount of the allergen. If you are intolerant to wheat or gluten, then chances are, you have been having symptoms for a really long time. Perhaps you think it is your norm to feel that way, or maybe you don't even know what it is that is giving you grief.

If you are having reactions like bloating, increased gas, indigestion, nausea or brain fog, to name a few, then you, my friend, are experiencing an upset in your digestive path, which is at one with your immune system. With all potential food intolerances, the only way to really know is to stop eating gluten for at least two weeks and monitor your symptoms, which can be a bit tedious, but hang in there. Keeping a food diary and noting your symptoms is also helpful, especially when you try eating it again.

Be aware, however, that when you remove a food group from your diet, you may find that the sensitivity to it is heightened when you eat it again. So, if you thought you could have a little bit of bread and you'd be OK, but you have avoided it for a length of time, eating it again may cause your symptoms to be worse than before.

With intolerances there is usually something going on behind the scenes. It could be that the person has a leaky gut or SIBO (page 129), and this is creating an overgrowth of bacteria and toxins in the body. Looking at solving the underlying issues can help heal or reduce the intolerance. Sometimes, though, it makes you feel so lousy that when you stop and feel better, you never want to eat it ever again, no matter how well you feel.

Because wheat and gluten can create inflammation in the body, it can be helpful to try it out. It can really help ease symptoms throughout your whole period career because cutting it out will help to reduce inflammation, and this can lessen symptoms.

I know some in the endo community feel fed up with hearing about how going gluten-free can help their symptoms. However, it has been found that cutting gluten from your diet for 12 months can decrease pelvic pain symptoms in 75% of those that have endo.[17] Got to be worth a try.

Coeliac disease

If you have coeliac disease, you absolutely can't have a crumb of gluten or any grain that contains gluten. It's another one of those diseases that often slips under the radar, but if you have a family member that has it, go and get yourself tested. If you notice that eating wheat/gluten affects you, then go and get a blood test. Interestingly, some can have irregular periods with coeliac disease, and there is a high chance that your inflammation markers will be screaming at you. I have worked with a few clients that have been coeliac, and we have found this out because when they gave up the gluten, they started to feel a whole lot different.

GLUTEN SWAP

Gluten-free (GF) food has come a long way since I first started my nurse training. Back then, the poor gluten-free patients had to eat bread that was like a breeze block!

There are lots of resources online to show you how to make or order gluten-free products. Supermarkets usually have a supply of GF breads that are pretty good. Some brands are better than others, so keep trying until you find what you like. I sometimes swap out toast for sweet potato – I slice them thinly and grill them, but you could even pop them in the toaster.

Be aware, however, that in terms of gluten-free cakes and biscuits, these will be higher in sugar. It helps them retain moisture, so it's added liberally.

The biggest thing to do when trying to cut out gluten is **read the labels!** It is in a lot of unsuspecting things:

Marmite, for example – I was so upset. Also, things like Worcestershire sauce (malt vinegar).

When reading the back of a packet to check if something is gluten-free, look out for the following: barley, bulgur wheat, rye, wheat, durum, semolina, brewer's yeast, malt, triticale, couscous and spelt, to name a few. Have a look at the Coeliac UK website (https://www.coeliac.org.uk/) for an extensive list because gluten is in a lot of things that aren't always obvious.

Oats are naturally gluten-free but get contaminated by contact with other grains – that is why there are gluten-free oat options. Buckwheat is also GF, even though it has wheat in the name!

MOOOVE OVER, DAIRY

The thing with dairy is the cows it comes from. Friesian cows are the black-and-white ones and the most common variety used. Their milk is high in A1 casein, which is a protein that upsets the apple cart of our gut and can set off inflammation.

If you are sensitive to this casein, you will have had – and may continue to have – hay fever, asthma and eczema, as well as ear, nose and throat issues. Casein can also contribute to heavier periods, more pain, PMT and acne.

Also, dairy is another food group that those with endo often benefit from avoiding, as this can help reduce their symptoms.

DAIRY SWAP

There are a host of different milks and yoghurts to try, from coconut to oat – just make sure they aren't loaded with sugar. Avoid oat milk if you are cutting gluten (because it can be contaminated by gluten). Also, make sure you aren't using ones that are mixed with vegetable oil of any kind –

these tend to be the barista-style products, or ones that they thicken up. You will see why in the next section. And finally, if you have oestrogen dominance tendencies (see Chapter 11), please swerve the soya products.

Organic milk from Jersey or Guernsey cows and dairy products from sheep and goats don't carry the A1 casein protein, so some find that they can eat this with less upset to their hormones.

Generally, with dairy, again, reading the labels is important because it can sneak in lots of places.

CHEWING THE FAT

The world of fats and oils can get very confusing quickly. We need a certain amount of fats in our diet to maintain health (other than trans fats, which we'll come to shortly), but it needs to be balanced. Fats can come from a variety of sources, including meat, fish, seeds, nuts, vegetables and man-made products (trans fats).

In terms of period health, the omegas are our focus – omega fatty acids 3 and 6, to be exact. Omega-3 helps to reduce inflammation as it gets converted into anti-inflammatory prostaglandins; omega-6 increases inflammation by creating more inflammatory prostaglandins. It's not as simple as saying 3 is good and 6 is bad – we need them both. It's just that we are exposed to a lot more of omega-6 in our food than omega-3, and that means the ratio is all out of balance. Addressing that balance – clearing more 6 out of our diets and upping our 3 intakes – helps us towards optimum period health.

In the blue corner, we have omega-3, which has three components: alpha-linolenic acid (ALA), eicosapentaenoic acid (EPA) and docosahexaenoic acid (DHA). We can't make omega-3 in our bodies, so we must get it through our diets or via supplementation. It helps to reduce inflammation, menstrual pain and the risk of heart disease and osteoporosis.

Omega-3 is found in seeds such as flax, pumpkin, chia and hemp, as well as avocados, walnuts, some alga, and eggs, meat and dairy from grass-fed animals. It's also found in fatty fish, such as mackerel, tuna, salmon, sardines, herring and shellfish, as well as in fish oil.

In the red corner, we have omega-6, which comprises of linoleic acid (LH). This breaks down to gamma-linolenic acid (GLA), which can break down further to arachidonic acid (AA), which is the component that kicks off the inflammation. It's found mainly in vegetable oils, which is most problematic to us because they are in EVERYTHING. Our western diet is full of vegetable oils, and they are found in processed foods, fast food, cereals, crisps, frozen pizza, confectionaries and milk alternatives. It is used to preserve food, cook food, make it more spreadable and stop it from caking. It sneaks in everywhere, and we are consuming too much of it.

Here is a list of the oils and the swap-outs you can make at home. Just doing this one thing can make a big difference. It's not to say you are OK to cook with a whole block of butter, but making some simple switches can really help to reduce the omega-6 in your diet and increase the omega-3. If you can get a hold of the cold-pressed varieties of the omega-3 oils, these are purer again. This is where seed cycling is also beneficial – see page 135.

Omega-6 oils/fats – *Inflammatory*:

- Sunflower oil
- Corn oil
- Safflower oil
- Soya bean oil
- Margarines

Omega-3 oils/fats – *Anti-inflammatory*:

- Avocado
- Butter
- Ghee
- Lard
- Duck/goose fat
- Rapeseed/canola oil
- Coconut oil *(doesn't carry omega-3s, but is a good substitute, as it's low in omega-6)*

Finding your balance here is key; it's not saying you have to have an all-or-nothing approach. Only eating omega-3s would not be good for you, as your body needs a mix of everything. I would suggest you start looking at the labels of things you have at home or buy regularly, and see if you can switch them out or reduce your intake of them if they have ingredients that are rich in omega-6.

Before I move on, I want to have a small word about trans fats. The World Health Organization (WHO) made a pledge to remove all trans fats from the global food supply by 2023,[18] but at the time of writing this book, billions across the globe are still unprotected from them.[19] There is nothing beneficial about trans fats, and they are to be avoided at all costs. It has been known since the 90s that they are detrimental to our health, in particular, to our hearts.[20] They are also wildly inflammatory to our bodies as a whole. Trans fats are partially hydrogenated oils, meaning vegetable oils (from the omega-6 list above) are combined with hydrogen in order to create a solid or semi-solid fat. They are found in a lot of different foods, including frozen pizza, microwave popcorn, some crisps, shop-bought bakery products, margarine, shortening, fast food and vegetable oils. You should read the back of packaging to find where it resides

Artificial sweeteners and sugar-free alternatives were wrongly seen as a healthier swap for sugar for decades, and fats have suffered a similar fate – turns out, full-fats from the omega-3 list above are actually good for us. Some dodgy deals and skewed data on animal fats and cholesterol have helped the rise of industrial seed oils in our diet and the fall of healthier natural fats.

CHAPTER 10 ROUND-UP

Being conscious of your food is a big win. It is overwhelming, this knowledge, and I apologise about the Pandora's box-type situation, because once you know these things, you can't unknow them! For now, though, I invite you to have a poke about in your cupboards and read the labels on your food. Just start to notice where all these food groups creep in, and where you can make some swaps. Taking little and frequent steps towards your end goals will make for the best and lasting changes to you and your body.

I don't think there is a one-size-fits-all diet. In fact, I know there isn't. On forums there is always hot debate on what works and what doesn't. The long and the short of it is that you will have to find something that suits you: if it makes you feel better, then it's working for you, and if it makes you feel below par or worse, it isn't. Sometimes, you are so used to feeling below par, you don't even know you are there until you start to weed stuff out of your diet.

It can look like this: cutting back on sugar suddenly gives way to more energy. It sounds ironic, but this stabilises blood sugars. You will then get better sleep, which reduces your stress and stops the need for sugary hits because your energy isn't through the floor. This, in turn, gives you the energy to try and get out for some walks or to the gym. So, the upward cycle of events starts to unfold.

There are lots of diets out there – low-carb, keto, paleo, vegan, the list goes on and on. To prescribe everyone the same thing won't work, it never does. As we age and our hormonal landscapes change, so do our nutritional requirements. In other words, your hormones need to be cared for by your nutrition. I see a lot of health coaches advocating a certain diet – usually low-carb – for perimenopausal women to help them maintain a certain weight. Concentrating on weight doesn't sit right with me. I want to concentrate on strength and vitality rather than aesthetics. I don't need a ripped tummy to be healthy; I also don't need to shed all of my body fat.

My diet looks like this – I'm gluten-free and 98% cow dairy-free. I will eat the odd bit of goat's cheese. I avoid processed food where I can, and I make 95% of my food from scratch. I invest in organic fruit, veg and meat where I can. I only eat chicken and fish – very fussy as to where it comes from, and if I'm eating out, I go vegetarian. I don't drink alcohol, and I don't eat sweets or milk chocolate, but I love dates and raw cacao, and I drink limited caffeine. I filter my tap water and use this for cooking and drinking. I use olive or coconut oil to cook with and have a little butter. I am still partial to a slab of gluten-free cake every now and then. I also promise I am fun to be around!

What the hell would you call this diet?! I call it 'what works for me', and it has been honed and tweaked over years. I am still learning, and I adapt to what my body needs as it needs it.

My clients find the food and nutrition part of supporting and balancing their hormones to be one of the biggest hurdles, largely because it's a minefield once you start poking around. It's one of the areas that we spend the most time on in My Whole Shebang wellness programme because it is a major player in our health. However, once there is a clear plan, and my clients start to feel better, the path to follow naturally becomes easier.

Following your body and its hormonal symptoms is the best way to find out what it is your body needs. Remember: all your hormones speak to each other, so if there are other aspects of your health that aren't tip-top, your period will help you discover them. You really have a natural health check every month, which is pretty crazy, to be honest, in a wonderful way. Aren't our bodies smart, considering how much negativity surrounds our hormones and how complicated it all is? Our bodies have complied by saying, 'OK, use this for information about our health.' I think this is a great way to reframe for those that have a dodgy relationship with their hormones and period.

END ON A POSITIVE

It's a lot, I know. This stuff isn't done in one fell swoop; it's little steps that build up to big changes. This sentiment is true for pretty much everything in this book *and* life, to be fair.

'So, what can I eat?!' I hear you cry. Remember the 80/20 rule: 80% on the straight and narrow, 20% wiggle room.

It's no secret – in fact, it's slightly boring. You need veggies, whole foods and seeds, and fruits for your sweet treats. You also need to be properly hydrated with water, not gin, and you should opt for organic foods where you can and reduce your processed food intake. Often it helps to have another set of eyes on what and how you eat, not for judgement reasons, but for a guiding hand to help you make better adjustments.

Sprouts, broccoli, flaxseed and maca root (a south American vegetable from the cabbage family) are some of the best food sources for helping the body excrete excess oestrogen. They bind to it and help oestrogen exit stage left. Making sure you stay well hydrated so you have good gut mobility, plus eating more fibrous veggies, will help with elimination, too.

Try eating breakfast if you don't, and if you are eating cereals and/or toast and jam, try changing it up and having a more protein-rich breaky. This will enable you to feel fuller for longer.

Eggs are a great source of protein, or you can try adding seeds and nuts to yogurt and fruit.

The best way to help yourself is to be ahead of the game. If you know you are in a rush in the mornings, have something ready you can grab made the night before. Slow cookers are the salvation for all busy households, as tasty nutritious food is made easy.

To become really intentional about your digestive health, keep a food diary and notice symptoms. These can only really be seen when you put awareness on them, or when you speak with someone who can guide you in understanding that what you are experiencing isn't something you have to put up with forever.

Food can also be used as a comfort and a way to numb difficult feelings and life events, but that shizzle will need to be dealt with before your reliance on cake, I'm afraid. We all have been in this place at some point or another. I just want to give you and your frazzled nervous system a hug and say, 'Please go and get some support – we all need it sometimes.'

The next section is going to look at oestrogen dominance and how we get extra oestrogen from some food groups and external toxic chemicals. This is an important piece of the puzzle when it comes to regaining balance with our hormones and endocrine systems as a whole.

CHAPTER 11

OESTROGEN DOMINANCE

If you don't see a clear path for what you want,
sometimes you have to make it yourself.

Mindy Kaling

The term 'oestrogen dominance' was first put out into the world by Dr John Lee in 1996. He believed that oestrogen dominance was the real issue behind our hormonal woes throughout our entire period careers. The term refers to our bodies having insufficient progesterone to balance out excessive amounts of oestrogen in our systems. Oestrogen dominance isn't recognised by doctors, so it might be better to talk about symptoms of overabundant oestrogen.

It's always worth saying that there is so much nuance around working with hormones, and nothing is black and white. Western medicine tends to subscribe to synthetic hormones to address an overabundance of oestrogen, and TikTok health gurus will tell you to do a celery cleanse

Both viewpoints do a drastic disservice to our intricate bodies and their wisdom. It isn't just oestrogen and progesterone we are working with here, but the entire endocrine system. We need to stop thinking we only have two hormones and start working with all of them, weaving the correctly patterned blanket for your exact requirements instead of just trying to smother everyone with the same one.

All of the reproductive hormones play parts in the overabundant oestrogen story. It's just that oestrogen and progesterone have the lead parts, and oestrogen is a diva. When these are all working well with each other, things run smoothly; when they don't, shit hits the fan. The script for your hormones relies on subtle feedback between your brain, ovaries and adrenals. Things like stress, diet, and exercise directly impact that conversation.

Oestrogen is the doer – it creates tissue growth. Progesterone is the project manager – it lets your body know when it's time to let go and reset. As much as oestrogen is made the big movie star, progesterone is its agent, keeping oestrogen in check, and helping your body break it down, metabolise it and get it out of its system. When oestrogen goes unchecked, it creates an imbalance in your hormones, and then you start displaying symptoms of having too much oestrogen.

This chapter explores what oestrogen dominance can look like, how it can occur, and how we can best support our bodies to redress any such imbalances which, in turn, can help regulate our cycles and reduce period pains and other unpleasant symptoms.

WHAT OVERABUNDANT OESTROGEN CAN LOOK LIKE

Overabundant oestrogen can be mild, moderate or severe. A blood test will also tell you if your oestrogen levels are particularly high. I am always a fan of getting bloods done because they can give you a benchmark to work with. Obviously, it can vary with hormone fluctuations, so working alongside your own symptoms is an excellent way to see your progress. I often get clients to write a list of all their symptoms when we start, and then they get the pleasure of ticking off the ones that disappear over time. There is nothing more satisfying than ticking things off a list!

Mild symptoms of oestrogen overabundance include:

- Premenstrual headaches
- Breast tenderness
- Fluid retention
- Menstrual cramps

Moderate symptoms of oestrogen overabundance are:

- Irregular menstruation
- Adrenal gland fatigue
- Heavy periods with clotting
- Dry eyes
- Hair loss
- Thyroid dysfunction
- Plus, the mild symptoms

Severe oestrogen overabundance may cause:

- Fibroids
- Endometriosis
- Breast cysts
- Adenomyosis
- Polycystic ovary syndrome (PCOS)
- Plus, the mild and moderate symptoms

HOW WE CAN BECOME OVERABUNDANT IN OESTROGEN

There's no single 'put your finger on it' answer to this, as is always the case with hormones and the endocrine system. However, there are some key triggers and indicators we should take a look at.

- **Not ovulating** – and therefore not producing progesterone, which counterbalances oestrogen
- **Low-fibre diets**, as we need fibre to keep our guts squeaky clean and pooing regularly; otherwise, our bodies will start to reabsorb toxins in our faecal waste if it's in our bodies too long, and this includes excess oestrogen the body is trying to eliminate
- **Stress**, since high levels of cortisol affect all our hormones
- **Environmental factors and using endocrine-disrupting products**

Overabundant oestrogen is likely a combination of all of these factors. When you are looking to help reduce the toxic load on the body, it's the small changes that can make the biggest differences. If you keep making those changes, bit by bit and over time, you will change a lot and start to feel better.

LOOK AFTER YOUR GUT AND LIVER

Your gut and liver health are big players when it comes to regulating inflammation and oestrogen overload. Your gut is thought of as your second brain, and it doesn't get that title for nothing. Your intestines' responsibilities include getting the goodness from your food. They are an integral part of your immune system, they communicate to the rest of your body via various substances and they serve as the body's waste disposal unit. Your liver has many jobs, but a key one is being the filter that metabolises drugs and detoxes your body of chemicals. It filters the blood from the digestive tract before it goes into the rest of the body.

If we are eating diets high in sugar, alcohol, veg oils, etc., as we discussed in the previous chapter; using products that disrupt the endocrine system (this is coming up); or depleting our bodies because we are stressed and not looking after ourselves – this ALL comes together and creates problems in the gut. In turn, the gut can't clear out the extra waste effectively, which contributes to running down our immune systems. This creates the perfect storm for increasing inflammation and can affect our hormones. Gut health is **vital** for hormone health.

The liver is astounding, too. It is one of the busiest organs in the body. It has the capacity to regenerate, and it puts up with a lot with very few complaints. I can't list all the jobs the liver does, but these are the pertinent ones to hormonal health. The liver...

- Metabolises fats, proteins and carbs
- Excretes chemicals and toxins (including excess hormones), cholesterol and drugs
- Stores glycogen*, minerals and vitamins

(*Glycogen is glucose that is stored in our livers and muscles. When we don't have enough glucose coming into our bodies via our food, or we need a quick boost of energy, we can convert glycogen from our liver and muscles. It is broken down and popped into our bloodstreams to energise our cells.)

I always make a beeline for the liver with every client I work with, as supporting this organ is a key part in filtering out the guff that doesn't need to be in our bodies. Imagine if you never changed the filter in a coffee machine – eventually you would get a scuzzy build-up of grounds. The same goes for our guts.

Ideally, our digestive systems should remain squeaky clean and full of good bacteria.

HOW TO TELL IF YOU HAVE UNHAPPY GUTS

If you are reading this and you know me well, you will know I enjoy a poo chat! No, we don't need to get out the kitchen sieve and go all out Gillian McKeith about it, but keeping an eye on what comes out of your body is important. Here are a few things to look out for when thinking about your gut health.

How often you go for a poo

Research suggests that having a poo anywhere from three times a day to three times a week is normal. Well, you know what I think about norms! There are lots of factors at play here as always: how much you eat and drink, what kind of foods you're eating, any underlying conditions, how performative your bowels are, etc. However, I would say changing things in your diet will have a direct effect on your bowel habits. Changes to them are important to note, because they are another point of communication from your body, and they signify how well your guts are.

When I worked as a nurse, I ate a diet of mainly beige food, was constantly dehydrated and worked shifts that made my body stressed. I didn't have regular circadian rhythms because I was always in a state of jet lag, so my bowels were slower than a steamroller going up Everest. Since having regular sleep, eating a better diet and keeping hydrated, I have a poo every day. Sharing is caring, but it goes to show how sensitive our guts are to our environments, inside and out of our bodies.

To my mind, every 24 hours is a good ballpark to work with (but if you have no symptoms and it's more or less, don't stress it). We don't want our waste sat in us for any longer than it needs to be because our bodies will start to reabsorb it and that is less than ideal. If your intestines aren't as efficient as maybe they could be, food can start to break down in the gut, rather than being put in the rubbish bin (toilet), and this can lead to other digestive issues.

Here are some gut-related problems that can have a direct effect on your hormonal health, so they're important to know:

- **Intestinal permeability** – This is when the gut is 'leaky' and allows what it is containing to enter back into the bloodstream.
- **SIBO (small intestine bacterial overgrowth)** – This is a condition that can get overlooked, but is essential to know. It is exactly what it says it is – bacterial overgrowth in the small intestine. It needs to be treated because it can cause malabsorption of nutrients. It's another reason we want great gut mobility, so rubbish isn't sat inside of us creating a breeding ground for bacteria. Symptoms include diarrhoea, nausea, weight loss and feeling full. It can be treated but it can also reoccur.
- **Yeast overgrowth** – When we think yeast, we think thrush, but we can have candida throughout our entire digestive tracts. When it is rife through the body, it can show up as very stubborn recurring thrush episodes. It should be a rare event, not something you see five times a year or more.
- **Coeliac disease** – I mention this here because I have worked with clients that have been diagnosed with this, and it's one of those things that can take years to diagnose. This is an autoimmune condition whereby those that have it can't eat a crumb of food that contains gluten. The delicate villi, which are hairlike structures that line your intestines, get damaged and malabsorption of nutrients becomes a problem.

Perhaps it's the nurse in me, still obsessed with fluid-balance charts, but I'm not alone in my thoughts on this. I agree the messaging is confusing, so it's why I am so passionate about us having agency over our health and symptoms. Although we have to take the perspective of everyone being different, a lot of functional doctors and dieticians agree that, ideally, our guts should perform once every 24 hours. Something everyone can agree on, though, is that stress affects our guts and makes them speed up their transit times, which goes to show the direct link stress can have on the body.

If you have no idea about what your gut mobility is like, keep reading because I have a little test for you!

> **Tip:** Drinking two litres of water a day really helps your toilet habits. The longer waste sits in your colon, the more water is sucked out of it, which can lead to stools that are hard to pass, so stay hydrated.

You are very windy and your farts leave others breathless

Another way to tell if your guts are unhappy is by way of your wind. If faeces is in your body for too long, it starts to break down and ferment in there. That can create some pretty lethal methane! Sometimes, it can be certain foods that give you gas, but it's also possible that it's caused by a sluggish gut.

Upper burps

If you eat something and start burping profusely a little while after, this can be a sign that you are putting something in your body that it's unhappy about. This can also be an indication of having low stomach acid right through to being coeliac. My point here is if you notice a pattern of eating something that repeatedly makes you feel uncomfortable, it's a tell that you can't tolerate it or your body is trying to communicate with you.

> **Tip:** Try the sweetcorn challenge! Sweetcorn hulls don't break down in your gut. They come out pretty much the same as they go in. If you eat a corn on the cob, and then start to look out for it in your stools, you will have an idea of how long food takes to work its way through your body.[21] Ideally, it shouldn't be in there for more than 24 hours.

Consistency of your stools

The Goldilocks of poo is 'just right' – not too loose and not rock hard. If you have constipation, it suggests food is sitting in the gut too long because you aren't drinking enough and your gut mobility is low. If you have rocket poos that are loose but you aren't unwell with a bug, this might suggest you have something stopping absorption, or there is an underlying condition that is upsetting your guts. Your hormones can also affect your guts – I'm sure a lot of us are aware of how we get increased poos as our periods approach, often thanks to prostaglandins. This is another thing to note when getting geeky with your body.

> **Tip:** Massage your tummy in a clockwise direction to help the peristalsis (movement) of your gut. You can go quite deep and firm. This can be helpful if you want to speed things along a bit.

Having a digestive system that works well enables you to clear out toxins more effectively. It allows you to metabolise efficiently and stop the body storing up things it absolutely doesn't need for later. It's no coincidence that the gut is called the second brain: it gives us a lot of clues as to the inner workings of the body.

Here are my top tips to help improve your digestive system:

- Drink plenty of water throughout the day.
- Make sure you have fibre in your diet, as this helps to chivvy along your waste.
- Reduce the toxic load on your system by cleaning up the products you use for yourself and in your home.
- Exercise, because it really helps your gut mobility to move your whole body.

INGESTED OESTROGEN

Oestrogen is a bit of a shape-shifter hormone. Unlike progesterone, which can only be produced one way, oestrogen is resourceful and has other ways it can form, both in and out of the body. As a result, we can be affected by it externally through our environment, as well as by everyday products and our food.

The types of oestrogen found in food are known as phyto-oestrogens. They are plant-based in nature and come in various forms, which we shall look at shortly. Consuming high amounts of these foods can and does make symptoms worse for those that have higher-than-average oestrogen.

The issue with the oestrogen in these food groups isn't simply that they have oestrogen properties; they can also be problematic because of the processes they have undergone or if they contain genetically modified or non-organic plants, i.e. plants covered in pesticides. After all, to produce a lot of food and make some money out of it, the cheapest options are always going to be used – and pesticides make harvests more lucrative. This is why, when possible, it's important to opt for organic.

BUT IS IT ORGANIC?

Being organic is a big deal. I know it's a privilege to buy organic because it's twice the price of regular products, so please do what you can with the resources you have. However, organic is important, and here's why.

Food is thy medicine; we are what we eat and all that, but really, food can be inflammatory to our systems, and it can add to the toxic load in our bodies. This is where being a bit more discerning about your diet is important.

A great way to find out the cleanliness of your fruit and veg is to check out the Dirty Dozen and Clean Fifteen. The Dirty Dozen are 12 fruits and veg that are likely to have high pesticide residue. These are:

1. Apples
2. Strawberries
3. Kale
4. Celery
5. Peaches
6. Grapes
7. Nectarines
8. Cherries
9. Pears
10. Tomatoes
11. Spinach
12. Bell peppers

The Clean Fifteen looks like this:

1. Pineapples
2. Sweetcorn
3. Avocados
4. Asparagus
5. Sweet spuds
6. Cantaloupe
7. Watermelon
8. Honeydew
9. Kiwi
10. Mangos
11. Cabbage
12. Frozen peas
13. Onions
14. Papaya
15. Mushrooms

Knowing these lists can help you make an easier choice on what to buy organic – or if you can't, what you'll wash thoroughly. These lists change each year, so do check: a simple Google search will give you the results.

TIP: Washing all fruits and veg thoroughly is worth its weight in gold. Soak them for 20 mins in a sink of water with some white vinegar and a sprinkling of bicarbonate of soda to help clean off any pesticides.

Eating foods with phyto-oestrogens can have an effect on the oestrogen you have in your body. Plant-based oestrogen is a weaker source of oestrogen, but can still result in changes to your hormonal health – some positive, some negative, depending how your hormones are to start with. Some phytos block and escort oestrogen out of the body, while others can boost oestrogen. Notice the symptoms of your period: have you started a plant-based diet, for example, and then noticed changes to your period? For some these changes might be positive; for others, maybe not.

Here is a list of the most common foods that contain phyto-oestrogens, with the top three being the most potent:

- Soyabeans/soya products
- Red clover (herbal medicine)
- Flaxseeds
- Legumes
- Pinto beans
- Alfalfa
- Chickpeas
- Brans

- Beans
- Fruits
- Vegetables

These aren't foods to be avoided, but you should be mindful of them, particularly the top ones. Soy is in so many foods that you can end up overdoing it by accident, rather than by design. Flaxseed, on the other hand, is amazing, as you will go on to read. This list is to help you make informed choices about your foods and see that by adding something as small as seeds into your diet, you can make a massive difference to your gut health, but also your hormones.

SEED CYCLING

Seed cycling can be a great way to help balance hormones. It is the practice of using seeds that are beneficial to the different halves of your cycle. For example, you would add pumpkin and flaxseed to your meals during your follicular phase, and make a point to eat sesame and sunflower during your luteal phase.

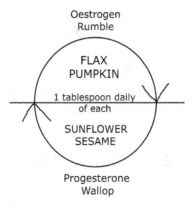

Oestrogen
Rumble

FLAX
PUMPKIN

1 tablespoon daily
of each

SUNFLOWER
SESAME

Progesterone
Wallop

Flaxseeds disrupt the enzymes that produce oestrogen and can help fill up the receptors, thus blocking toxins and excess oestrogen from getting in the receptors.

Flaxseed is high in omega-3s and amazing for the gut, and if you are prone to constipation, it helps in that department, too. Be sure to purchase whole flaxseeds – pre-milled tends to be less fresh, in my experience – and whizz them up in a coffee grinder. You can then store them in your fridge for a couple of weeks. A dessert-spoon's worth a day is ideal. Just keep in mind that, if you have issues with higher oestrogen, flaxseed does carry oestorgen properties. Generally, I would recommend using flaxseed in your diet, as it helps to clear out toxins in the body by binding the excess oestrogens and removing them. Having good bowel movements is another way to detox!

In my experience, soya is one of the more problematic phyto-oestrogens, mostly because it has been used to replace A LOT of food groups, especially in a plant-based diet, for example. It features in most food groups, and the phyto-oestrogen effects of soy are cumulative in the body over time. If you are displaying symptoms, and you are eating a lot of soya, try cutting back on it or cut it out completely for a couple months and see if you notice anything different with your periods.

Phyto-oestrogens are a great asset to our health, easy to weave into our diets and can have great effect on the body. They can be really effective at helping detox our bodies and regulating our hormones alongside other aspects of our health.

XENO-OESTROGENS

The oestrogens that come from our environments, homes and personal products are known as xeno-oestrogens. These don't actually have oestrogen in them, but contain chemicals that mimic oestrogen (affecting women and men), and they disrupt our endocrine systems, even in minute concentrations. These chemicals latch onto the body's oestrogen receptors and fill up cells, making more oestrogen in the body than it would produce naturally.

Avoiding xeno-oestrogens isn't something we can do completely nowadays, and you could become neurotic trying. But there are things you can put in place, small changes that can make a BIG difference. This is another Pandora's box moment, I'm afraid, and most of us are marinating in a toxic soup, to some extent – I fear for those working in the perfume sections of the duty-free airport shops. I literally can't breathe in those places!

'Xeno-oestrogens' is an umbrella term for thousands of chemicals that have oestrogen-mimicking properties, and here are some of the common ones:

- **Parabens** – These are used to prolong the shelf life of make-up and personal body-care products.
- **BPA (bisphenol A)** – This is found in polycarbonate plastics and epoxy resins. Polycarbonate plastics are used in containers that store food and beverages, such as water bottles, and epoxy resins coat the inside of food cans, bottle tops and water supply lines to our houses.
- **PFAS (per- and polyfluoroalkyl substances)** – These are known as 'forever chemicals' because they don't break down. PFAS comprise a selection of 12,000 chemicals mostly used to make thousands of products resistant to water, stains and heat, such as Teflon, for example.
- **Phthalates** – These are fragrances found in perfumes, air fresheners and any fake scent added to something like soap, shampoo or washing powder. They are used in plastics that need to be flexible and not break.

Xeno-oestrogens are found in the following products, and this is by no means everything!

- Pesticides, herbicides and fertilizers
- Some deodorants and anti-perspirants
- Shampoos and skin creams
- Most sun creams
- Fuels and car fumes
- Polycarbonate plastic bottles, including some babies' bottles
- Plastic food containers
- Cling film/tin foil
- Inside of tin cans
- Fragrance

Here are the top five things you can do to help remove environmental toxins from your life and home right away:

- Take your shoes off in the house. It's such an easy win because you pick up a lot of environmental toxins on the bottoms of your shoes that you don't want in the house.
- Open your windows daily to let fresh air into your home.
- Avoid synthetic air fresheners.
- Soak your fruit and vegetables in a vinegar and bicarb solution.
- Vacuum and wet dust regularly.

All cells have receptors on them like mini cups. Some of our cells have receptors for different hormones. These fill up with the stuff that enters our bodies and goes into our bloodstreams. If there are lots of endocrine-disrupting chemicals in our bodies, they fill up these cups and upset the balance of oestrogen in our bodies. We have oestrogen receptors in our breasts, uteruses and thyroids. Helping to reduce the toxic load we put on our bodies helps to reduce the risk of excess oestrogen in our systems, which, in turn, helps us to reduce period and hormone symptoms.

If you think that big companies have your best interests at heart, think again; instead, their lack of concern can often lead to products being less than beneficial to your health. The Johnson & Johnson baby powder scandal – in which asbestos was found in talc, and links between cancer and the product were uncovered[22] – is up there with how diabolical big corporations can be. Please don't ever use baby powder. If you need talc, use corn powder. Another example is the research that has come out about the effect of chemical hair straightening and its link to uterine cancer.[23] This predominantly affects black and brown women who tend to use these products more often.[24]

Science has known for years that something is afoot with our endocrine systems due to the amount of pollution we are ingesting and living in. A study that collected 30,000 umbilical cord blood samples found PFAS in **every single sample**. Links have been made between these foetal exposures and health complications in unborn babies, young children and beyond.[25] PFAS exposure in the womb has also been linked to a lower sperm count in males.[26] These chemicals are changing us, making us sick and affecting our fertility, and most of us have absolutely no idea.

When I first started figuring stuff out with my own cycle and periods, I looked into my period products. I used to use whatever was on special offer, usually the big commercial brands. Looking into this further, I was horrified to find out I was sitting on the equivalent of four plastic bags in each pad. The cotton in both the pads and tampons was bleached and doused in chemicals, and the companies that make these products aren't required to put the ingredients on the packets because they aren't considered medical products.

I switched to reusable pads and a menstrual cup and, for the first time in my life, my cycle started to become regulated; it also was less painful. I could not believe it – and I could not wrap my head around the fact that I had never questioned the vulva pillows I used every month. I assumed they wouldn't be bad for my health because of the very nature of what they are.

I am so pleased to see a massive boom in reusable period products on the market nowadays. Please, if you do just one thing, only use organic cotton disposable pads or tampons, or get involved with reusables. You are not only helping the planet, but you are helping your body. Also, don't put your tampons down the loo, please – they have to scoop them out of our waterways, along with sweetcorn and gravel, the latter of which I hope isn't anything to do with what we eat!

CHAPTER 11 ROUND-UP

Your health matters. Brené Brown said that if women stopped buying personal and beauty products for a week, it would bring the industry to its knees. I won't lie – I would love to see that happen.

As with it all – balance, balance, balance. You can drive yourself crazy with learning these things if they are new to you. Your hormones can be affected in many and multiple ways: by your diet, products and your internal and external environments. Be your own detective and start reading the labels to see if you want to continue using something knowing it has a host of chemicals in it.

All these factors come together to create a perfect storm that can contribute to painful, problematic periods and menstrual issues (and their knock-on effects). Follow advice given in this chapter, and it will help. And get to know yourself via charting and general body literacy, as this is the key to everything.

And above all, do small things often, as this amounts to a lot. Rome wasn't built in a day, and neither will your chemical-free lifestyle.

CHAPTER 12

PLANTS! AS MEDICINE?

The best time to plant a tree was 20 years ago;
the second-best time is now.

Chinese proverb

Plants predate pills – that's it, end of story, case closed. We used plants way before paracetamol came in a pink box just for periods. I had a mixed reaction from people when I decided to study plant medicine, especially as a nurse. Considering one of the biggest plants out there allows us to breathe, I would say that they deserve quite a few kudos! How plant medicine came about fascinates me – it's just wild to think how many people would have died trying to find out what works.

'Where's Dave?'

'Oh, he's brown bread. He ate the berries before they were fermented in the light of the full moon and stirred anticlockwise for three days with a mammoth tusk.'

'Shit.'

My belief is that health is two sides of the same coin; there is Western medicine and then there is everything else. There is room for both, and I wish we could work together more – the results would be fantastic. I see the benefits of the inventions and technology we have – I'm sincerely grateful to have anaesthetic rather than having to bite down on some leather! However, in terms of women's health, modern medicine can often fall a bit short.

In this chapter, I will be covering some history behind plant-based medicine and going through some of the common herbs used in herbal medicine, plus sharing some blends of my own that can be helpful to support you.

A BIT OF HISTORY

Ancient Greek physician Hippocrates was first to discover that white willow bark (*Salix alba*) had pain-relieving qualities. It was the precursor to aspirin because it has salicylic acid in it. This bitter compound, found in some plants, is what aspirin is made from to this day.

Science got excited about the idea that certain chemicals could be isolated and extracted from plants. However, when they extracted *only* the salicylic acid from white willow bark to give to people, it led to internal bleeding. Why? Because in its natural state as willow bark, the other chemicals in the plant balance out the acid's effects.

Next to be tried was meadowsweet (*Filipendula ulmaria*), which also contains salicylic acid. If was found that meadowsweet could help with pain relief but also protect the gut at the same time. Plants are intelligent like that.

The pharmaceutical company Bayer managed to synthesise what we know as aspirin and went on to trademark acetylated salicylic acid (synthetic salicylic acid). They put a lot of energy in marketing how acetylated salicylic acid was gentle on the stomach, and the natural, plant-based alternatives dropped in popularity.

Plant medicine isn't a new thing; it's been used for thousands of years. Archaeologists have found the practice of herbal medicine can be traced to as far back as 60,000 years ago in Iraq. Our ancestors risked a lot from strange poisoning accidents to glean the knowledge we have now. I like to honour that sacrifice by learning a craft that is ancient and also increasing in popularity again.

Our bodies have innate wisdom, and we are interconnected to nature whether we like it or not. In all my training in alternative therapies, I have always kept an open mind. Having medical training can sometimes be a blessing and a curse! For me, I always want to get to the root cause of something, not band-aid it. The band-aid approach is the go-to management technique for a lot of chronic conditions in medicine, especially in terms of women's health. This gap is also down to a lack of research and funding. I fully suspect most medications that we take in our everyday lives have never been tested specifically in relation to how they affect our menstrual cycles.

CASE STUDY ON HERBS

When I first started working in alternative therapies, I did wonder in the back of my mind if they were going to work. I worked with my first client, who had endometriosis, over several months, and she got to the point of having pain-free periods. I had never seen such a smile on someone's face – it was something that she hadn't experienced before. Watching the changes my clients make and seeing the positive outcomes never fails to bring me huge job satisfaction. It also proves the power of alternative therapies, time and time again.

WHICH HERBS CAN HELP YOU?

I urge you to explore all of your options when working out how to best care for your periods and hormones, so you make any decisions through informed choice. There are many valid options out there, and making decisions when you are desperate or frustrated is never the best – but I know how easy it is to get to that place! Most of my clients arrive at my door feeling hopeless about their situations, and I love nothing more than seeing all that start to turn around.

It can be overwhelming trying to find out which herbs can help you. When I work with clients, I tend to use blends that are specific to them and their needs. Before we take a look at some of the individual properties of some of the kickass herbs I use, I'd like to give a general overview of the ones that can help with specific hormonal issues.

I always advocate working with a herbalist – herbs are medicine, after all. The information coming up is for your own reference, and you can do more research if you wish. Working with a herbalist will always offer you more specialised and tailored care. I generally work with these herbs in a tincture form. They can be found in specialist shops in powders and tablets, but tinctures are the preferred way to administer, as they have a higher concentration and they can be blended with other herbs. Some herbs, it's fair to say, taste disgusting, so you wouldn't want to drink them in a long drink like tea.

Below, you'll find a list of period-related issues, as well as the herbs that can help remedy them.

Painful periods:

- Burdock (*Arctium lappa*)
- Chaste tree (*Vitex agnus castus*)
- Cramp bark (*Viburnum opulus*)
- Milk thistle (*Silybum marianum*)

Heavy periods:

- Chaste tree (*Vitex agnus castus*)
- Lady's mantle (*Alchemila mollis*)
- Milk thistle (*Silybum marianum*)
- Stinging nettle (*Urtica dioica*)
- Yarrow (*Achillea milefolium*)

PMS:

- Ashwagandha (*Withania somnifera*)
- Chaste tree (*Vitex agnus castus*)
- Milk thistle (*Silybum marianum*)
- Skullcap (*Scutellaria lateriflora*)

Endo/adeno:

- Burdock (*Arctium lappa*)
- Chaste tree (*Vitex agnus castus*)
- Myrrh (*Commiphora myrrha*)
- Turmeric (*Curcuma longa*)

PCOS:

- Ashwagandha (*Withania somnifera*)
- Chaste tree (*Vitex agnus castus*)
- Milk thistle (*Silybum marianum*)
- Turmeric (*Curcuma longa*)

Perimenopause:

- Chaste tree (*Vitex agnus castus*)
- Milk thistle (*Silybum marianum*)

- St John's wort (*Hypericum perforatum*)
- Wild yam (*Dioscorea villosa*)

Menopause:

- Black cohosh (*Actaea racemosa*)
- Chaste tree (*Vitex agnus castus*)
- Milk thistle (*Silybum marianum*)
- Red clover (*Trifolium pratense*)

YOUR HERBAL HEROES
Chaste tree (*Vitex agnus castus*)
This is a herb that's special because its only effects are on the female reproductive system. It works on the pituitary gland, balancing out your hormones, including the luteinising (LH) and follicle stimulating (FSH) hormones. It helps with regulating prolactin and prostaglandins and it's something I use with my clients a lot.

Cramp bark (*Viburnum opulus*)
Excellent for period cramps, this herb helps the uterine muscles to relax. It also helps to support the nervous system, increases circulation to the muscles and can regulate heavy bleeding.

Burdock (*Arctium lappa*)
A great herb for digestion, burdock promotes healthy gut bacteria and regulates inflammation. It is also excellent at getting toxins out of the body. A powerful antioxidant, it protects the liver and stimulates bile production. It can also be helpful to use for acne because of its detoxifying properties.

Milk thistle (*Silybum marianum*)
Considered a brilliant herb to support the liver and digestion, this fab antioxidant helps to protect the gut from inflammation. It also boosts immunity and prevents free-radical formation.

Stinging nettle (*Urtica dioica*)

The stinging nettle is one of the most well-known herbs we have growing in the UK, and it's also found across the globe. Nettles are powerful when it comes to strengthening and supporting the whole body. They have astringent properties that help to relieve symptoms of heavy bleeding.

Lady's mantle (*Alchemila mollis*)

This herb helps to regulate periods and is good for supporting progesterone production. It helps stem heavy bleeding and is a powerful astringent, and can also alleviate period cramps. It can be used in the peri and menopause to help balance hormones, and also supports the gut and can be beneficial for skin health.

Yarrow (*Achillea milefolium*)

This is an excellent herb to stop bleeding when placed on a wound, as it increases the clotting action. Useful for those with a heavy periods, it helps to tone the muscles of the uterus, which improves menstrual flow. It is also a great herb for those that have amenorrhea (absent periods), and it supports the digestive system.

Ashwagandha (*Withania somnifera*)

This herb supports the immune system. It also helps the heart and can stabilise blood sugars and cholesterol levels. It is a great adaptogen herb, meaning it can energise and calm at the same time, depending on needs of the body. It is helpful in supporting the reproductive system.

Skullcap (*Scutellaria lateriflora*)

One of the most widely used and well-known nervine tonics, skullcap helps to relax the nervous system as well as renewing and reviving it. It's great for those who are exhausted.

Myrrh (*Commiphora myrrha*)

Myrrh has excellent antibacterial effects on the body. It's also a powerful anti-inflammatory, which helps to ease pain. Useful in supporting the liver because it detoxifies and has high levels of antioxidants, it also supports the kidneys and helps to excrete toxins. It is a key herb for endo and adeno.

Turmeric (*Curcuma longa*)

An antioxidant-rich plant, turmeric is excellent for soothing inflammation in the body. It also boosts the immune system and helps to protect the heart and brain. Black pepper helps to activate turmeric, so they are best used together.

St John's wort (*Hypericum perforatum*)

Most known for its antidepressant properties, this herb also helps to lower cortisol and support the body's nervous system.

Wild yam (*Dioscorea villosa*)

Wild yam helps to relax muscles and support the nervous system. It can also help with balancing hormones.

Black cohosh (*Actaea racemose*)

A good hormone balancer, black cohosh can be helpful for symptoms like night sweats, hot flushes, mood swings and anxiety. It helps to ease cramps and regulate periods, improves uterine tone and has anti-inflammatory properties (salicylic acid is present in this herb). It also aids nerve function in the body and reduces nervous tension.

Red clover (*Trifolium pratense*)

Red clover has flavonoids, which are a phyto-oestrogen. It can be helpful during the menopause and can support heart and bone density. It also helps to reduce any depression and anxiety associated with the peri and menopause, as well as being good for the skin and respiratory system.

Incorporate the right herbs

As you can see, herbs can do so many wonderful things in our bodies. This is why it's always best practise to work with a herbalist, so they can work with the specific requirements of your body and give you the herbs you need.

It is also fair to say I am not of the opinion that using herbs alone is going to fix all your problems. They are part of the toolkit to help you heal – one aspect that, together with all the other things in this book, can make a massive difference.

MAGNESIUM

Magnesium is a beaut of a supplement to get on board for your period health. It is very helpful for the ol' cramps. You can take supplements and use them alongside the herbs. Another way to get involved with magnesium is with Epsom salt baths... heaven! Or you can make a spray using equal parts Epsom salts to water – use boiling water to dissolve the salts, allow the mixture to cool and bung it in a spray bottle. Spritz all your fleshy bits with it every morning and evening.

MY BLENDS

Herbs can work well on their own but are often stronger together. I have a whole load of speciality blends that I have lovingly put together with hormonal issues in mind. I've blended my herbal potions so you get the best of all the herbs out there. Herbs can be taken in various forms, the most common one being an alcohol suspension; you will typically take a teaspoon of it orally at least twice a day. Alcohol is the popular choice because of its preservative properties, which provide longevity. You can also turn herbs into a tea. Although their effect isn't as strong in this form, it can be a great way to incorporate them into your daily life. Vinegar is also used as a suspension sometimes, but it isn't so common.

Here are a couple of examples of my blends so you can see how the herbs can work together.

FUCK THAT SHIT

This is my number one blend for helping support the nervous system. Anyone that is feeling fatigued, anxious or burned out needs to get involved with this blend, which is fantastic for supporting the adrenals and helping to balance cortisol in the body. Because stress can create imbalance for our hormones, this is a really helpful potion for supporting your nervous system. Oats and wild yam have qualities in them that support the menstrual cycle as well. Herbs generally have the capacity to work on more than one system in the body – they are very clever like that. This blend also comes with a healthy affirmation in its name! Fuck that Shit contains the following:

- **Oats** (*Avena sativa*) – Oats are one of the best remedies for feeding the nervous system when it is under stress. The seeds and/or aerial parts of the plant are used. It works on the nervous system and is a real nurturing herb. It can help with exhaustion and support other herbs that are helping the nervous system, so that's why it works so well in this blend. It helps to strengthen the nervous system as well as support it.
- **Siberian ginseng** (*Eleutherococcus senticosus*) – This herb is great to help increase stamina when we're facing extra demands and stress, be that physical or mental, it's all the same to our bodies. It's great for exhaustion, depression and helping the body find its resilience.

- **Skullcap** (*Scutellaria laterifolia*) – This is one of the most widely used and well-known nervine tonics, and it helps to relax the nervous system while also renewing and reviving it. It's great for those who are exhausted, and it gets bonus points for being helpful with premenstrual tension.
- **Wild yam** (*Dioscorea villosa*) – This herb helps to relax muscles; it's really good at easing the muscles in the intestinal tract and helps to support the nervous system as a whole.

BITCHING

This is my PMT potion and it helps to iron out the symptoms we can experience during the lead up to our periods. It contains:

- **Chase tree** (*Vitex agnus castus*) – This herb helps to balance and restore order with our hormones.
- **Wild yam** (*Dioscorea villosa*) – As well as relaxing muscles, this herb also gives a bit of balance to our hormones. In particular, wild yam supports the progesterone end of things, which is what can so often be overshadowed by oestrogen.
- **Chamomile** (*Matricaria chamomilla*) – This herb has a gentle sedative effect and is helpful for reducing inflammation in the body. It also helps to support the nervous system and reduce pain.
- **Black cohosh** (*Cimicfuga racemose*) – This powerful herb helps to relax and normalise the female reproductive system. It supports painful or delayed periods and is very good for cramps and cramping pain. In general, it helps to balance hormones, reduce nerve pain and relax the nerves.
- **Mugwort** (*Artemisia vulgaris*) – Mugwort is a bitter tonic that helps stimulate the digestive system. This is important because it helps to clear toxins out of the body and ease

tension. It is also a tonic for the nervous system and aids the regulation of menstrual flow.

If you would like to find out more about how to buy my herbal products or work with me, details can be found at the back of the book.

CHAPTER 12 ROUND-UP

As with nutrition, and all the other chapters in Part 2, this one is aimed at supporting you and your body, not in isolation, but as part of a holistic approach to your health and menstrual health in particular. I hope it gives you some food for thought and things to try!

CHAPTER 13

EXERCISE

Be a badass with a good ass!

Our bodies, brains and nervous systems thrive on exercise. It is how we humans have always connected with our environments: by moving through them with all of our senses. A new concept for many, however, is the idea that we should be aware of where we are in our cycle when we exercise, and change what we do accordingly.

It's important to look at why we want and need to move our bodies. Forever, the narrative has been to get thin and ripped, but that isn't a healthy goal. Moving your body is about building dense bones and strong muscles to support the skeleton, providing stimulation for the brain, relaxing through movement and getting the feel-good chemicals going. It also improves our overall health and helps us maintain a healthy weight for us – but the weight thing is very subjective, and all body shapes benefit from movement.

The exercise we choose to do will, to some extent, automatically change depending on our cycles, energy levels, the time of day, our sleep patterns, and what we have or haven't eaten. We aren't machines doing the same things day in day out. Variety is important, and working with our bodies and getting joy from what we do is important, too.

We are all in different places, and where we are in life also creates boundaries. Just popped out a baby vs having teenagers vs being kid-free – different people are going to have a different mix of time and energy. This doesn't always mean new mums are time-poor and those without kids have all the time in the world. The patriarchy would have you believe things were all linear like that and tied up in a nice, neat bow of toxic productivity. That just isn't how it works when you have a menstrual cycle. Nothing is straight – it's always a circle.

I have a love-hate relationship with exercise, and I have tried loads of different things to find what I enjoy the most, because the key word in that whole sentence is ENJOY. Without that there is little to no hope of sticking to anything. The pandemic really did a turn on my fitness, and it highlighted how much I needed it in my life and how much I missed it. So, all of you out there reading this and sighing right now, I feel you – I'm talking to myself here more than anyone else!

In this chapter, we'll look at the importance of exercise, some exercise hacks and inspo, the key muscles of the pelvic floor, and some specific advice in relation to exercise and your period.

WHY IS EXERCISE IMPORTANT, AND WHAT'S IT EVER DONE FOR ME?

Exercise is good for all aspects of your health and well-being – there is no denying that **not** moving your body is very bad for your health. Leading a sedentary lifestyle isn't healthy, mentally or physically. It's never too late to start getting into the swing of things, though.

'Use it or lose it' is a pretty accurate slogan when it comes to fitness and mobility. Your body morphs itself to whatever you do most – think how athletes' bodies are shaped by what sport they do. When we are babies and young children, we are like rubber bands in terms of mobility, but as we age, this changes. Chairs are a big part of the problem. Throughout Asia, for example, it is really common to see all ages squatting as they watch the world go by or chew the fat with a friend. In the West we don't squat like that – a lot of us would fall over in about a minute. Our bodies are used to chairs; we haven't comfortably used the squat position in that way since we were probably three years old.

There is, as ever, a balance to be struck with all this. You don't want to be booming and busting with your activity, like a bull in a china shop, and then feel unable to move. Moderate and steady wins the race on this one. Remember: exercise stimulates the nervous system, so honouring your cycle and working with that can help you pick the right exercise for you. It might need to be a kick-ass HIIT (high-intensity interval training) workout, or it might need to be a more relaxing yoga class, for example.

Going 0–60 at a million miles an hour increases inflammation and weakens the immune system. Ad hoc activity where you beast yourself and then don't do anything for days puts more stress on the body. Moderate, regular activity, on the other hand, boosts the immune system.[27]

Getting outside in nature to exercise gets extra points – it has greater benefits for our health than training indoors, it releases the good chemicals in our brains that make us feel better, and our stress levels drop.[28] Being outside, we activate that ancient part of ourselves, the one that got all its information from the environment, not Google.

As well as clearly being good for our overall health, regular exercise also has the following benefits, all of which can particularly benefit menstrual health. It is good for:

- Improving confidence
- Improving posture
- Increasing energy
- Reducing the risk of osteoporosis

- Potentially helping with easier childbirth
- Improving flexibility
- Helping reduce anxiety and stress

Let's dig a little deeper to look at some of the benefits to our bodily systems – in particular our hormonal health and landscape – and where there are some overlaps.

- **Hormones** – Exercise has a direct impact on our all of our hormones. Activity of all kinds helps to release dopamine and serotonin, for example. But studies have found that exercise changes hormonal output, which alters our metabolism so we can meet the needs of the activities we are doing. This is a very complex mechanism in the body.
- **Brain** – This might not seem pertinent now, but heading into our perimenopause and menopause, brain health becomes significant. There are many studies that conclude that exercise reduces the risk of age-related brain disease. Getting hot and sweaty helps with the neuroplasticity of our brains, but our modern way of living can severely reduce that capacity, and the consequence of that is our brains age quicker.[29]
- **Bones and muscles** – Exercise builds strength and, again, this is a bit of a future-proofer for the peri and menopause. There is a vital window in the transition between the two worlds of peri and meno, which is difficult to predict: the last two years of your peri and the first two years of your meno. This is when big changes happen with your hormones shifting around. Building a strong body before that window helps you through it. It's within that window that bone and muscle loss are at their peak. I will talk more on this in the peri and meno chapters.
- **Flexibility** – As babies, we could touch our toes, no problem, but we tend to lose this ability by sitting too much. It's so important for our back and pelvic health to be

flexible, so stretching and flexibility should always be part of an exercise session (if not the whole session).

- **Mental health** – This is directly related to the ability of exercise to reduce stress which, in turn, has a positive impact on everything else. The reason it's so good for us is because it brings out the endorphins, the body's happy hormones. That high can be very addictive, which is my only explanation for why people keep doing marathons!

BUILDING A STRONG HOME FOR YOU TO LIVE IN

Moving our bodies in a variety of different ways is important. Take an elite swimmer or runner, for example. They won't *only* swim or run to build their fitness; they will do a whole load of other things that all come together to support their body as a whole.

Ideally, we should be attempting a mix of strength, aerobic, balance, flexibility and mobility training in our exercise. These different areas look a little like this:

- **Strength** – Basically, these are things that make you say *oofft*. Think: lifting, pushing or pulling weights, or using your own bodyweight, too.
- **Aerobic** – This would be something that makes you blow out of your arse a bit, the runny, jumpy, mind-your-knees stuff.
- **Balance** – Truth be told, balance comes into all exercise types. Concentration is needed so you don't look like one of those inflatable things outside car sale rooms with their arms flailing everywhere!
- **Flexibility** – Yoga and Pilates-type movements allow you to stretch and free up your body and keep it supple. It's a really important aspect of movement, and can help you stay healthy.

- **Mobility** – This is something you get in all types of exercise, but it's sneaky because there will be things you could do when you were younger that you think you still can, and turns out, no! Mobility isn't just walking around; it's the mobility of your body – maybe your ankles or hips, for example – and isolating the places that are stiff and need a bit of work. Usually, mobility issues happen because of a weakness in muscle/strength in one area, so other muscles or joints jump in to compensate.

I'm no expert on exercise, so I asked Samantha Sands, a personal trainer, for advice, and she said this: 'I've been working in the fitness industry for ten years. There are always new ideas and concepts, but consistency is the key to it all. It's so important for women to be fit and strong. There are no down sides, only positives.'

EXERCISE DURING YOUR PERIOD

For some of you, exercising during your period will be OK, and for others, it'll be a hard no. However, some **gentle** exercise can help with many symptoms, such as:

- Pain/cramps
- Bloating
- Mood swings
- Irritability
- Depression
- Fatigue

You have never needed to tune into your body more than at this time though, because when it comes to your period, it is very much in the driving seat! Exercise can be great, but you must have the energy to start with. Don't push yourself, and remember: it's all about balance.

EXERCISE TO TRY

The following are exercises you might want to get involved with when you are on your period.

- **Stretching** – Yoga and Pilates can be fabulous when you have your period, but you might want to pick the more easy-going classes, or Nedra or restorative yoga.
- **Walking** – This is such a good all-round activity, and you don't need to have special equipment or a membership to anything. You can also change up the pace as you see fit.
- **Aerobics** – I couldn't even contemplate running during my period, but if you fancy a little jog, go half as hard as you normally would. You can also try a swim or bike ride, but don't push yourself.
- **Strength work** – Be led by your body, and don't overdo it. After you lift, try some gentle stretching into the areas you feel you need it most.

Doing nothing is also valid; always remember, **resting is doing something**. Your body is bleeding – that in itself is quite a big physical event. So, supporting that by not doing anything is 100% valid. I, myself, am a big supporter of the do-nothing approach. When it's bleeding, I think my body is doing enough already. A couple days off exercise won't hurt anything; always be led by your body at this time.

EXERCISE TO AVOID

There are some types of exercise I would definitely recommend avoiding during your period, namely anything strenuous or workouts that might involve inversion.

Strenuous exercise

So, I think that rules out bungee jumping, rollerblading, parachuting and any other adventure sport they have shown on period-product adverts! Doing hard-core physical activity during your bleed can increase inflammation. If you are someone with a heavier flow, you might also see an increase in bleeding with strenuous exercise simply because you are shaking everything around. And increased inflammation also brings the increased risk of pain. If you have conditions like endo, adeno fibroids or heavy bleeds, I will give you a permission slip every month to miss PE when you have your period.

Inversions

It is advised in the yoga community to skip inversions (head stands and legs up the wall, etc.) while you are bleeding, as your energy is coming out of your body. You do you, but listen to your body – highly likely it wants it feet up on a couch, rather than in the air!

If you buy into the 'no pain, no gain' mentality, you will find no support for it here. Pain is a signal to STOP, always. If you try any exercise during your period and you feel pain, nausea, fatigue or dizziness, stop. And don't come back until your period has fully finished.

RELAXIN

Relaxin is a hormone that is released during your cycle. During your cycle, you have two relaxin peaks: one during your period and the other during ovulation. It is those times when injury can occur because you have less stability in your skeleton, basically. This lends more importance to knowing where you are in your cycle, which allows you to better work with your body. So, it is difficult to give you a time frame of days here because it will depend on your cycle, but I would ballpark a couple of days around ovulation, as well as during the most active part of your period.

Relaxin is something we associate with pregnancy mostly; it is present throughout pregnancy and is released by the corpus luteum and then the placenta. What happens the majority of the time is that progesterone and relaxin work together to thicken the uterine lining. If no pregnancy occurs, both hormones reduce, and a period happens. You need to know that you will have a spike of relaxin at ovulation time, which then dips and peaks again during your luteal phase till your period – and this is a time to be a bit more wary about doing funky stunts at the gym.

If you have had a baby, you may have heard about relaxin because its effect is to make the cartilage and ligaments of the pelvis looser. This can lead to symphysis pubis dysfunction (SPD) – but the thing is, it works on all cartilage and joints, not just the pelvic ones! SPD is a condition that creates pain in the pelvis. It can happen more often in the later stages of pregnancy and can make walking and moving around very uncomfortable.

EXERCISING AND LEAKING

It should come as no surprise to say that there is more chance of blood making a bid for freedom if you are moving around more. I say, if in doubt, wear it all! The adverts lied – no amount of wings are gonna cut it for the heavy bleeders out there, unless there are a lot of toilet stops.

Regardless of how your period rolls, there is no escaping the extra fanny admin it requires. There are great products out there to get involved with – the period pants are a particular win. I would double up on my protection: pants and pads, or cup/tampon plus pads. It just gives you some peace of mind.

Dark clothes are helpful – remember the recent uproar at Wimbledon when the women mentioned that it might be nice not to have to play tennis during their periods in full white regalia?! Or you could get a yoga mat like mine that has a massive fake blood stain right in the middle of it. I bought it like that – *CSI* eat your heart out, no one would ever know! I must say, though, no one has ever asked me about it, and I'm a little sad about that!

YOUR PELVIC FLOOR

This is the hammock-like muscle that supports your uterus, bowel and bladder. All of your openings to these parts of your body go through your pelvic floor. I think it's fair to say we only hear reference to it in terms of it not being tight enough after having humans, which is a bit sad. It is a big part of women's health to look after and nurture your pelvic floor, so it should get a bit more attention than it does really. We can hold a lot of tension in this area, and I feel education about the pelvic floor is a bit sparce. I hope this gives you some pointers.

POSSIBLE CAUSES OF A WEAK PELVIC FLOOR:

- When you have had the most Olympian workout of them all – pushing a human out of your loins
- Extra weight during pregnancy
- Obesity
- Chronic constipation
- Straining to poo
- Constant coughing
- Surgery that requires cutting the muscles of the pelvic floor
- Reduced oestrogen after menopause
- Recurring pelvic floor muscle tension caused by painful periods or endometriosis

We all know the one about sneezing and wetting our pants. It's something else that has been normalised – they even sell pads for it, FFS! – but it shouldn't be.

WHAT A WEAK PELVIC FLOOR MIGHT LOOK LIKE:

- Leaking urine when coughing, running, sneezing or laughing
- Not making it to the toilet in time
- Passing wind from the anus and/or vagina when lifting or bending
- A heavy sensation in the vagina
- Dragging and/or heaviness in the pelvis or back
- Recurring urinary tract infections
- Recurring thrush
- Vulval pain
- Pain during sex
- Inability to orgasm
- Reduced sensation in the vagina
- Tampons that escape and fall out

PELVIC FLOOR EXERCISES

Doing regular pelvic floor exercises is important. Ideally, they need to be done every day from puberty onwards. Squeezing this group of muscles is no different than working out any other muscles in your body, and strengthening them will be future-proofing your pelvic health. Having an awareness around your pelvic floor also helps you use those muscles when you need to, during exercise, sex and childbirth. Some dos and don'ts:

- Do quick pulses – aim for 15 pulses and repeat 10 times.
- Don't stop yourself from having a wee mid-flow – that's just asking for cystitis.
- Do engage your pelvic floor muscles when you cough or sneeze.

POSSIBLE CAUSES OF TENSION IN THE PELVIC FLOOR

Surprisingly, women can sometimes have issues with their pelvic floor because the muscles are too tight – and not in a good way. This can be caused by:

- Doing a lot of fitness and holding in the core – not allowing the muscles to have some downtime
- Holding it in and not going for a wee and/or poo – I'm talking hours, as sometimes people feel uncomfortable going to public loos
- High levels of stress – part of the fight or flight response makes us tuck in our tail bone, which puts tension on these muscles

WHAT TENSION IN THE PELVIC FLOOR MIGHT LOOK LIKE:

- Pelvic muscle pain – this is the most common symptom and is generally always present
- Pelvic pain
- Constipation/straining when emptying the bowels
- Not emptying bowel completely
- Urinary incontinence
- Incomplete emptying of the bladder
- Urinary urgency
- Urinary frequency
- Painful urination
- Slow flow of urine
- Hesitancy or delayed start of urine stream
- Lower back pain
- Hip pain
- Pain in the coccyx, the bone at the base of your spine
- Painful sex
- Vaginismus

To help yourself with tense pelvic floor muscles, you need to be seen by a pelvic physio. Gift yourself an appointment, as getting that sorted out can be life-changing. We don't have to just accept incontinence or prolapses as part of ageing or having kids. We can take the control and get back in the driving seat. If more education was given on protecting our pelvic floors, we probably wouldn't see so many problems. Knowledge is power – never be embarrassed for asking questions. Just because they sell incontinence pants, doesn't mean you have to use them. Sorting out the underlying problems would be a better solution, which is possible and will set you free to sneeze and laugh with gusto.

FINDING WHAT WORKS FOR YOU

Exercise has been lumped into the 'eat less, move more' category, as if this is the holy grail of health. It is seen as a tool to reshape our bodies and make us trim and beach-ready, whatever the hell that is.

I tend to grab my swimmers for the beach, not my abs, and if I can get away with it, I prefer to be starkers anyways! I think the emphasis on appearance and results has made a lot of people fear exercise and see it as a chore when it's something that can be fun. If we take the pressure off doing it for any other reasons than making us feel good and having enjoyment, it would seem a lot less scary, and I reckon we would be more up for giving things a go.

To me, exercise is a feeling, I might hate it at the time, but afterwards it feels bloody brilliant and everything about my day is much better. I like to exercise with others; particularly, I like to have a buddy to keep me accountable, and with whom I can share my sweat, tears and wobbly bits jiggling around, and celebrate afterwards.

There are so many things to try – the list is rather endless. Regardless of what you choose, please look after your knees in all that you do! I cringe sometimes in classes I have attended when there is no proper warm down, or they are making people do squats and lunges at super speeds. Please ALWAYS listen to your body. Yes, pushing yourself at times is a good challenge to take on, but that needs to be done at a pace and time that works for you. Injuries can knock us off our perches for a while.

Doing something every day for five minutes will do more for you than exercising once a week for an hour. Breaking things down like this makes it all less overwhelming, and you can take time to build habits and work things into your personal routine. You don't have to get ready for it, either; just go from where you are, you deserve to feel amazing. I cheerlead those that feel shy about fitness the loudest – it is for ALL of us.

You don't need to look at the trendy accounts on social media for inspo; you don't need abs or a tan, the best trainers or long, flowing hair – you need to love your body and get out there and give it what it needs, which is a whole lot of love.

SOME THINGS TO TRY:

- Treat yourself to a personal trainer for their expertise and accountability.
- Tune in to freebies that are available online.
- Join a gym to sample a variety of new classes and see what you like.
- Make a commitment to meet a friend to exercise.
- Get off a stop earlier and walk to work if you take public transport.

And take a look at the following list for some suggestions of things you can cultivate that might further inspire you on your exercise journey:

- **A good workout playlist** – Put one together with all the songs that inspire you. You can't tell me I'm the only one to have a full 'Eye of the Tiger' moment while working out when it comes on the headphones!
- **An encouraging mindset** – This is a key part of the whole picture. Talking yourself out of exercise is easy, right?! So, if we can do that, we can talk ourselves into it.
- **Accountability** – Ask a friend to help keep you accountable, and to maybe come with you.
- **Pride in yourself** – No one looks amazing while working out. As we do during sex, we pull a varied number of faces and makes noises that we have no control over when we exercise! There is nothing to be embarrassed about, so don't let the risk of farting when picking up a weight put you off!

CHAPTER 13 ROUND-UP

No one is born ripped – they all have to work at it. And, personally, that isn't a look I aspire to, but to each their own. We all have to start somewhere, and those steps are usually small ones, but with time and by picking something you enjoy and having the right cheerleading squad about you, you can literally achieve whatever you want. I will say it again for emphasis, too – **you do not need to visit the gym in order to wear a bikini or go to the beach.** You already have a beach body, a beautiful body, and anyone you allow to touch it should be very grateful indeed.

As your body ages and changes, it needs different things, and movement can be used to attain this. But what worked for a bit might not continue to work now, and that is more than OK. On the flip side, with continued practice, what you might not have been able to do, you now can because you have allowed your body to grow in strength and resilience. You have the capacity to achieve so much.

What would you like to achieve? Can you write down some goals towards which you would like to work? One of mine was to be able to do a full push-up – I got there eventually and I felt chuffed!

CHAPTER 14

I CAN'T STRESS THIS ENOUGH

*Emotions are like waves, we can't stop them from
coming but we can choose which ones to surf.*

The dictionary definition of stress is 'a state of mental or emotional strain or tension resulting from adverse or demanding circumstances.'[30]

We can't live without stress, and to try to avoid it at all costs is neither sustainable nor achievable. Life has other plans, and it can feel like we are living in a continuous mercury retrograde at times! However, the nervous system is designed for short bursts of stress, not for us to be habitually living in it ALL the damn time.

To understand stress, we have to understand the working of it in our bodies, which is essentially a manifestation of our fight, flight or freeze response. Not very sexy, but we can't override this – it is a response as old as time. As I remember Ruby Wax putting it, 'Your brain is designed to keep you alive. It doesn't give a shit about your feelings.'

You might be wondering what this has to do with your periods. Well, quite a lot, actually. If you go back and look at Chapter 2, you will see that our adrenal glands pump out adrenaline and cortisol. These two hormones have a direct effect on your overall health which, in turn, has an impact on your period health. You can't be releasing lots of one hormone without it having side effects on the rest of the endocrine system.

Stress is one of the biggest things I work on with my clients. Their stress might come from their periods themselves, or it might be from other aspects of life but still impact their period health. It's no accident that my best-selling potion by a clear mile is Fuck that Shit, which is used to help with anxiety, adrenal fatigue and stress. We are all feeling it and generally lack any skills to get a handle on it, and antidepressants aren't for everyone!

So, before we look at the effect of stress on our bodies, let's look at the whole process.

THE FIGHT, FLIGHT OR FREEZE RESPONSE

Our brains are so sophisticated – and ridiculous. We have two parts of our brains: the lizard side, which is like a Nokia 3210, and a new brain, which is like the latest iPhone. These two halves of our brains have grown together but both kept their respective software. The Nokia is wired to the past, making nano-second judgements by sorting through previous experiences, always working on keeping us safe and not giving a flying fuck about our happiness, I may add! The iPhone part, as we all know, is always getting upgrades if we want them, by learning, reading and having therapy; it has neural plasticity which means you *can* teach an old bird new tricks. We can change thought patterns, learn new things and build resilience to things we only dreamed of. This is exciting, but it takes continued practice and repetition because our lizard brains will have tantrums as we step outside of what it deems our safety zones. It will try and herd us back to what we have always known, which can cause us to feel a little stuck. So have faith – it's OK to feel a bit like Bambi when we try things for the first time and we're being vulnerable, wholehearted and brave.

Stress is an umbrella term for leaning into our fight, flight or freeze (FFF) response. It's ancient – it is how we have survived thus far. We either ran away from the tiger, fought it and killed it, or froze and hoped it didn't see us. We don't have literal tigers to face anymore, but life can throw us metaphorical ones left, right and centre. As such, our reactions are still the same as if we faced a real one, and all the same stress responses happen in our bodies. This response is part of the autonomic nervous system (ANS), and we have no control over it, which is a good thing – we would most likely forget to breathe if it was left to us to remember! The ANS sorts out involuntary processes such as breathing, blood pressure, squeezing the heart 60 times a minute, digesting food and getting turned on. The ANS is broken down into three branches, but the ones we want to look at are the sympathetic and parasympathetic nervous systems. Now, I always have found the best way to remember this is by the irony that the sympathetic nervous system alights when you are in FFF, and the parasympathetic is in action when you are chilled, as you are whilst reading this.

You CANNOT be in two places at once with this – you are either stressed or calm – but things can also change rapidly. Think of kids' parties: everyone is having a great time until someone gets so wired they end up biting someone else! Excitement and anxiety can feel the same in the body. I say to my clients that it's like anxiety is confused excitement. And our thought patterns can influence how we feel about a situation.

Some people are so accustomed to their stress and anxiety levels that they become high-functioning. Their outward appearance is that of a swan serenely gliding along the water, but underneath they are paddling madly.

SYMPATHETIC AND PARASYMPATHETIC NERVOUS SYSTEMS

Let's take a look at what happens in your body in the two different parts of the automatic nervous system.

Sympathetic – Your inner meerkat

Your sympathetic nervous system kicks in when your body feels it's under any kind of threat. It looks like this:

- You're on high alert.
- Your digestion stops.
- You are looking about the place.
- You have a short fuse.
- Your blood pressure, breathing and pulse go up in anticipation of something bad happening.
- Adrenaline and cortisol floods your system.

This is your body in survival mode, living hand-to-mouth, and if it is a permanent state of affairs because of stress, it is quite unsustainable and very costly to your health and well-being. It also has a direct effect on your hormonal health.

Parasympathetic – Cool as a cucumber

On the other hand, your parasympathetic nervous system is where you hang out most of the time. Here are the signs that is has kicked in:

- You're digesting food with ease.
- Your blood pressure, breathing and pulse are within normal ranges.
- You can be still.
- Oxytocin and endorphins float around our body.
- You're able to relax and have a much more open demeanour.

When you are operating from your parasympathetic system, you are much more resilient, and you are able to acknowledge your stress and choose how to deal with it, perhaps walking towards it or away. Ideally, you are in your parasympathetic most of the time, popping into sympathetic periodically and then returning back again. There is a varying spectrum that you slide along with stress. Things like meditation, exercise, orgasms, laughing, hugs and pets can all positively enhance our placement on the stress sliding scale.

This is what I mean when I say you can change your behaviour and thoughts. Exercise is one of those things for a lot of people where the devil on their shoulder will tell them to sack it off, whereas the angel is saying it will be good for you, help you relax, etc. It can be a real struggle to get going sometimes – you know the angel is right but the devil's advice is so much easier!

As I said before, people can present as calm on the outside and still be stressed. These people are known as high-functioning stress-heads. They think they have it all under control, but ignoring stress is like trying to keep an angry octopus in a box: legs escape every now and then and wallop them around the chops. In other words, hiding stress makes matters worse. Let's have a look at how.

CHRONIC STRESS

Acute bouts of stress happen and can be good for us. For example, acute stress can trigger us to take action on getting an assignment done that we've left to the last minute – guilty as charged! But prolonged stress is harmful to our bodies and minds, not least because it results in serious hormonal imbalance. So, how can you tell when you are chronically stressed and living in a constant state of adrenaline soup? Stress can manifest as any or all of the following symptoms:

- Feeling exhausted
- Feeling irritated – and quickly
- Headaches
- An upset stomach
- Disrupted sleep
- A weakened immune system – feeling unwell all the time with colds, cold sores, mouth ulcers, etc.
- Procrastination
- Worrying constantly
- Finding it hard to concentrate
- Withdrawing from others
- Having low self-esteem and feelings of worthlessness

Stress can be also seen as an increase in some or all of the following behaviours, as we try to hide from our problems:

- Regularly getting take-outs
- Drinking more booze
- Falling asleep on the sofa in front of the TV
- Doom-scrolling
- Smoking
- Trying to complete eBay, aka overspending

How many of these can you relate to? Are you feeling them all month long? Or are these feelings more intense at certain times of your cycle?

YOUR INTERNAL HEALTH-AND-SAFETY MANAGER

As discussed, in perceived or actual danger, our brains trigger our sympathetic nervous system, so we will either fight it out, run away, or freeze and hope they don't notice us. This has worked well for us for millennia, but notice how I said 'perceived' as well as 'actual' danger. I did so because our brains can't discern between what is real and what isn't – hence why horror films scare the pants off us, even though we are watching in the safety of our own living rooms.

It's clear that being in survival mode puts a big strain on our bodies and well-being. It is not a place to hang out often. We might be so used to operating in survival mode that we don't even notice it. Stress can manifest into bigger versions of itself – anxiety and depression can all stem from unaddressed stress that is left to go feral.

Things that have happened to us in the past can also create FFF responses, and we might not even know what the trigger was or is. It could be something that happened in childhood or something we have blocked out or won't acknowledge. Humans are adapted to deal with things in many peculiar ways, except perhaps the most obvious, which is to address them. Patterns of behaviours are created in childhood, and these then play out throughout our adult lives.

Getting a therapist on board is often a suggestion I make to a lot of my clients, because mental health is key to developing the skills to love ourselves enough to look after ourselves. Healing this stuff takes time, but we need to bring our minds and bodies together to do so. We can't *think* ourselves well, we have to *feel* ourselves well. What I mean by this is, we can have the knowledge and understanding of something about ourselves, but to really understand it we need to look at what our bodies are doing. There are usually discrepancies between what we say and what we do, but if we can link those two things together, that's when we start unlocking the parts of ourselves that might not make sense to us. We don't need to remember what happened; we just need to feel the resistance our body has, then we can start to work with it. Our bodies know way more than we give them credit for. We can learn to sink into our inner marshmallow of wisdom, and it is a sweet place to operate from.

GET TO KNOW YOUR GREMLINS

Remember: the lizard brain is all about unconscious decisions set on keeping us safe no matter what, so it creates lizard gremlins that live and grow inside of us. These can manifest into negative thoughts or fuel existing ones – like 'I'm not enough,' 'I don't know what I'm doing,' 'They are much better than me so I won't bother,' 'I will never find love,' 'I'm not worthy.' There are tons of the little fuckers, and they hamper our progress because they are just like the actual gremlins from the film. They are delinquents that are awful to you – they are mean, they are rude, and they don't like change. It's up to us to really treat them like the toddlers they are. Sadly, an awful lot of them are generational, meaning they have been handed down to us through our families, and/or we are told or modelled behaviours and patterns. The really crazy thing is we often aren't even aware of it, this stuff needs a therapist. Please do that for yourself – it is the best investment you will ever make. In the meantime, though, challenge these thoughts. Would you ever speak to a friend the way you speak to yourself? I highly doubt it! Speak to yourself kindly, do it out loud if you have to, and tell the gremlins to fuck off, they aren't welcome at your table anymore. The gremlins are bullies, so stand up for yourself and let loose on all the things you have always wanted to say but didn't. It will have you fist-punching the air, and actually, if you keep going and get a bit ridiculous, it will make you laugh.

We do need some stress to get things done and over the finish line, but the trouble is many of us have normalised this high level of stress as the place we hang out most of the time, and that has burnout written all over it. Toxic productivity has a lot to do with this as well. For example, we seem to think we have to respond to that text now, this very minute, otherwise the world will end – remember, we used to write letters as correspondence!

LEARN TO FINISH THE STRESS RESPONSE

Something else that isn't linear is the stress response. We generally don't finish our stress responses, and so they get encapsulated in our bodies. It's so important to get that shit out! If we were being chased by a lion and it suddenly dropped dead, we wouldn't just stop running and think, 'Oh well, that was lucky, I'll just carry on picking berries.' We would most likely need to carry on running, shout our heads off, punch something – probably the lion! Actions like these would complete the stress response.

If we didn't (or don't) do this, we would (or will) have so much adrenaline flying around our systems! We need to shift it from our bodies, and the only way to do that is to expel it with moves like the ones I described above. Think about how athletes sometimes roar when they complete an event. That's it, that's the full cycle being completed. Imagine not finishing an orgasm – I think we can all relate to how that would feel janky AF.

If you own a pet, watch how they behave during the trip to the vet. All their stress responses come into play: they are calm getting out the car, then it builds as they enter the building, panting, pacing and whining. When you leave, they shake themselves – they are actually shaking off adrenaline. They are completing their stress response – a reset, so to speak – and they can then carry on with their day, forgetting the experience until the next time! Animals also get the gist of always living in the present.

Shaking your body is a great way to release adrenaline. It can be a full body shake, or maybe just the hands and feet, but it is important to see that whole process through. Otherwise, it actually gets stuck in the body, and that can create problems.

Now let's take a look at how all this impacts our hormonal landscape...

STRESS AND OUR HORMONES

Having looked at the nature of stress in our bodies, how it works and why it isn't a place we want to dwell, let's jump into what this means specifically for our hormonal well-being.

Stress and hormones are a match *not* made in heaven. Stress does a number on your whole body – there isn't a part that isn't affected by it – but hormones are especially sensitive. Stress can cause hormone imbalances, disrupt cycles, stop periods, lower libido and affect fertility. Do I have your attention?! It increases the body's inflammation markers, and it depletes our immune systems. It squeezes our adrenals dry, puts pressure on our insulin consumption and then sends our blood sugars into a spin. All of this has a knock-on effect on our hormonal health.

We've already met adrenaline and cortisol, the two main hormones released when the body is stressed. To recap, adrenaline and cortisol are break-glass-in-case-of-emergency hormones – they aren't meant to be lived on consistently. Our adrenals are the small glands that sit on top of our kidneys, and they pump out adrenaline and cortisol when needed to kick us into FFF mode.

If we operate under a high level of stress all of the time, it starts to change how our other hormones talk to each other. High cortisol in our bodies can affect testosterone, oestrogen and progesterone production. It can cause testosterone stocks to be depleted and oestrogen levels to be lowered. A depletion of testosterone can lead to the following symptoms:

- Abnormal periods
- Weight gain
- Muscle loss
- Joint pain
- Insomnia

- High cholesterol
- Reduced libido
- Osteoporosis
- Infertility

And decreased oestrogen can cause:

- Irregular periods
- Weight gain
- Hot flashes
- Night sweats
- Fatigue
- Mood changes

Progesterone is particularly sensitive to cortisol. In fact, cortisol is the biggest roadblock to progesterone being made because the body will not ovulate if it doesn't feel safe, and being in survival mode tells the body it isn't safe. Our bodies are very clever.

Low progesterone can look like:

- Headaches and/or migraines
- Mood changes
- Anxiety
- Weight gain
- Depression
- Reduced libido
- Sore boobs
- Problems with ovulation
- Irregular periods

Other areas in the endocrine system that are affected by stress include:

- The thyroid – the building blocks of metabolism

- Hormones that regulate appetite – 'stressed' is 'desserts' spelt backwards, after all
- Melatonin – hello, insomnia
- Insulin – insulin resistance and erratic blood sugars give rise to hangry moments

All of these areas feed into a vicious cycle, playing into each other and offsetting other areas until eventually we collapse in snotty heaps on the floor, harshly judging our life choices.

Overall, the hormonal changes that come from this little lot and relate to our cycles can cause:

- Changes in cycle
- Irregular periods
- Changes to flow/length of periods
- Fatigue
- Mood changes
- Weight changes, up or down
- Anxiety and/or depression
- Hot flushes
- Night sweats
- Vaginal dryness
- Insomnia
- Decreased libido
- Hair loss/thinning
- Skin tags

LOOK AFTER YOU!

Problems arise when you are stuck in chronic patterns of stress, or you don't care for yourself properly during the stressful life admin you can't avoid. I'm not laying blame here, but I am saying that most of us are ill-equipped to manage our stress. Feeling guilty for setting boundaries, or not doing so at all DOES NOT SERVE YOU. The naff sentiments of pouring from empty cups and fitting your own oxygen mask are there because they are TRUE! You can't outsource your needs to others – it doesn't work that way. They can only be met by you: you knowing them, acting on them and helping others to understand them. You don't have to be a dick about it, but you do have to turn up to the practice, and it might make your ass sweat to set boundaries, and that is more than OK. Sermon over.

LIVING OFF YOUR ADRENALS IS NOT COOL

Remember that the hypothalamus and pituitary gland are the all-seeing eye of your hormones. Activation of the hypothalamus-pituitary-adrenal axis is a prominent neuro-endocrine response to stress, promoting survival. What this means is living from your adrenals consistently creates a pretty clear message to your endocrine system and your nervous system that you are in danger and therefore living in survival mode – which means the bare essentials for your body and health. You CANNOT thrive in survival mode, but our Western culture, society and working environments often put this way of living on a pedestal.

Hypothalamus–pituitary–adrenal axis dysregulation (HPA-D) aka adrenal fatigue

Adrenal fatigue isn't always recognised by science, but I very much see it and believe it. And the reason I mention HPA-D is because of the domino affect it has – not on just our physical and emotional resources, but also with the inflammation it creates in the body. As we already know, periods are inflammatory events, and having extra inflammation in the body creates issues with them, increasing pain and volume, for starters.

HPA-D destabilises our blood sugars, which sets off a chain of events that cause us to crave all the wrong foods. We want quick hits of energy and all the processed carbs. However, low blood sugars actually activate our adrenals, so we end up in some terrible dance between the highs and the crashes, eating crap and creating more strain on these important glands.

We can't care for ourselves in the best way when we are feeling this depleted. Everything is extra heavy and that feels overwhelming, so it's hello, large glass of wine and cake to numb it all away. Sleeping becomes an elusive beast, cortisol interferes with our melatonin, and we feel too tired to move our asses to help shake off some of the adrenaline. We keep doom-scrolling and all that blue light buggers up our melatonin even more!

Some of the signs and symptoms of adrenal fatigue are:

- Feeling mentally and physically exhausted
- Waking up when in bed
- A buzzing head
- Not falling a sleep until the wee small hours
- An inability to get going till about 9am
- Crashing at about noon and then again about 3pm
- Feeling exhausted before crawling into bed and then lying there like you have taken speed
- Needing all the sweets and carbs to keep going
- Living on caffeine
- Feeling unable to exercise because of all the above
- Having trouble concentrating
- A failing immune system – getting all the bugs going
- Feeling unable to cope with stress

If you think you're suffering from adrenal fatigue, there are some things you can do to help yourself:

- Stop taking your phone to bed with you.
- Sleep in the dark.
- Cut back on the stimulant drinks – caffeine and booze.
- Dump the processed foods and swap them out for wholefood alternatives.
- Cut back on the sugar.
- Practice some deep breathing – in for four, out for eight, in reps of ten.
- Get out in the daylight and walk in nature.
- Keep a worry journal to help you see your thoughts.
- Eat regularly – don't skip meals and defo don't skip breakfast.
- Set a regular bedtime.
- Delegate jobs where you can.
- Start taking my Fuck that Shit potion.
- Rest, rest, rest.

CHAPTER 14 ROUND-UP

The stark reality is that we are all dealing with trauma – with either a little or big T – from childhood, adolescence and into adulthood. It's there in all of us. I think there is a shift happening and a recognition that we need to heal all parts of ourselves for health to be achieved. It's time to let that past trauma go and allow yourself the gift of freedom from it.

There is NOTHING that will heal your emotional landscape externally – it has to come from within, and you have to sit with your gremlins and set some ground rules. It's tempting to wallow and leave the responsibility with others. If you know you have a gremlin that needs dealing with but you refuse to go there, it is going to keep you trapped and in an uglier place with it, to be honest. Remember in the film *Labyrinth*, when Sarah says to the Goblin King, FINALLY, 'You have no power over me'? That's where you want to get to. All these negative nellies that reside in you only have power over you if you let them.

Again, I repeat, **getting therapy is such a gift to yourself**. And getting a therapist that you gel with is also crucial. Then, you can off-load that weight, cough up the emotional furballs that may have done what they needed to do when you were younger, but now need to be put to bed.

It's boring though, I get it, being told to fix your stress, eat healthy and move your ass, which may as well be topped off with 'and smile more'. We are all in the same boat here, we are smart cookies, and we know this shizzle. The big question is, why don't we do it? Our emotional health and well-being are intrinsically tied to our physical health and well-being, but we also want the silver bullet, the quick fix, and health most of the time takes a bit of a scenic route. It's been a scenic route getting to this place, a whole lot of ignoring things until they are unbearable, and then a scenic route out. The cha-cha-cha of health and well-being: two forwards, a couple sideways, but ultimately always moving forwards.

CHAPTER 15

YOUR FRAME OF MIND

Life's not fair, is it? Some of us drink champagne in the fast lane, and some of us eat our sandwiches by the loose chippings on the A597.

Victoria Wood

Following on from all that stuff about stress, let's look in more detail at how you can train and exercise your mind to better support your general health and well-being which, in turn, will support your menstrual health.

HELP, MY MIND IS FULL!

I'm a trained mindfulness teacher, and part of my training was spending a week in a Buddhist monastery, sometimes in silence. I may have laughed a lot during the silence – I'm only human – but it changed my life.

Mindfulness is non-religious, but you can see where it gets its inspiration. It is all about bringing awareness to our everyday lives: all our tasks, our breathing, eating, sex, work, walking, talking, the lot! And what that awareness does is make us fully present with our surroundings and experiences, rather than chatting with a friend but really thinking about something at work, or watching the TV but being on our phones, with nothing getting our full attention. Being mindful means we are fully immersed in something – such as learning a new skill, doing a creative task or even exercising – and are so engrossed that we don't think of anything except what we are in the process of doing.

A core practise of mindfulness is meditation, and one of my favourite meditations is bringing myself back into my body. We spend most our lives in our heads, when there is a lot of wisdom in our bodies that we miss out on. Meditation is not always easy, and it's one I've struggled with, but that's why it's my favourite.

When I suggest meditating with my clients, I am quite often met with cries of, 'I can't, my head is so busy,' 'It's hard to sit still,' 'My mind is full!' My advice is always to start small and build up to it, because your brain is a muscle, and like working out any muscle, it's something that will get stronger with practise. If the thought of sitting still for five or ten minutes is daunting, try building up to this in small increments that will take you just over a week. Here are some pointers to help you get started:

- Set reminders on your phone. There are apps you can use to set random or fixed-time reminders.
- Start off by sitting quietly and doing 30 seconds of breathing in (through your nose) for a count of 4, and out for a count of 8 – that's about 3 sets.
- Notice how you feel before and after the exercise.
- Increase by 30 seconds each day until you are cruising at 5 minutes of a simple breathing meditation.

Such a simple technique can feel difficult to start with, and then you wonder why it wasn't always in your life! Your breath is one of the easiest things to focus on but you could also notice the rise and fall of your chest or belly as your breath enters and leaves, or notice the pauses that happen between breaths. I also suggest the Calm app to my clients, which has a lot of resources, including guided meditations, that can also be very helpful when starting out.

Studies have shown that mindfulness meditation lowers the cortisol levels in the blood, suggesting that it really can lower stress.[31] And lowering cortisol and stress will have a knock-on effect in managing the impact these things have on your period health. It might not happen overnight but, over time, it will have a massive impact.

By focusing on the here and now with mindful meditation, you are not focussing on your thoughts. They will try to intrude, but if you return to focussing on, say, the breath, they will pass by. Thoughts aren't facts – they are just a collection of stuff passing through your brain that are signals as to how you are feeling, an overall radar on where you are in the world at that moment. Most of what you think about isn't true, it's assumptions you make about your perception of things.

The aim of meditation isn't to stop thinking all together – it's to turn it down, quieten the chit-chat and bring some calm, like turning down the volume on your internal radio so it becomes background noise. Sometimes, it's harder than others, and that's OK. In fact, even when you have been doing it for years, you have bad days at it. Come back and try again later – just don't use that as an excuse to not do it at all!

When you meditate you access different brain waves, and this can allow for some ideas to flow. If I get a great idea in my head, I will write it down; otherwise, I will just be thinking about that the whole time – then I can get back to meditating.

SHAKE IT OFF

Comedy has been one of the strangest teachers to me about all this stuff. I find I relate a lot of things back to it because the energy work involved with an audience is a lot! I've died on my ass practising my craft, but as much as it smarts, it's nothing compared to my thoughts about everyone who I think will be judging me. Yep, it's uncomfortable to watch someone struggle, it's uncomfortable to struggle, but no growth happens without it. In hindsight, I know no one is talking about that now, they probably weren't even talking about it when they left the club – we are all so caught up in our own stuff, people don't notice half the things you think they do. Use this to your advantage, go forth and be kick ass! I also use comedian Sarah Millican's rule: I give myself until 11am the next day to feel crap or great about how a gig went, and then I move on so the energy isn't trapped in me to affect the next effort.[32] I'm shaking it off!

I CAN'T SIT STILL THOUGH!

Cortisol and adrenaline (see Chapter 14) make you fidget – it's part of being in your sympathetic nervous system. That's why starting small and building up in terms of mindfulness meditation is important. Your body will want to rebel against sitting still. You can do mindful walking, which can be helpful, as can listening to a guided mindful walk. As I said previously, giving your body a good shake to let go of the adrenaline can be a good shout, as it completes the stress cycle. Or doing a meditation after exercise can also be an optimal time for fidget bums. Sometimes, you are going to have to sit with that discomfort until it softens, and you can let it go. It's also OK to stop, do something else and come back to it, as long as you do return because meditating helps to bring you back to your parasympathetic place. After all, one of the biggest benefits of meditation and yoga is that they help bring awareness to the breath, which is a really key element to helping you refocus and calm down.

I actually have my own power playlist on Spotify. I've curated tunes that create good vibes only, have banging beats and/or uplifting lyrics, and nourish my soul. I encourage all my clients to create a unique playlist of their own. Again, lots of studies have found listening to self-selected or classical music to be beneficial after something stressful has happened, not least because it helps us to complete the stress response if we move with it.

HAVING A MINDFUL CYCLE

I put this into practice and created a course called 'Unflappable – How Not to Lose Your Shit with Your Period'. It contains meditations for your cycle and gives you a meditation for each season. It can be really helpful to use something that reminds you of where you are in your cycle, what your body might need and your energy capacity at each point!

I thought it would be fun and helpful to have something to work on, specifically with the cycle in mind. My focus is very much on bringing the listener back into their body and remembering the wisdom that resides there. You pick the meditation that coincides with the season you are in and listen to that daily for the time you are there, then move on to the next one. You will find it easier to know your season if you chart and also trust your intuition.

I have included one meditation in this book but have made it more generic so it's useful at all times! This is a great one to bring yourself back into your body so that you can check in with what it is you might need today. I have used nose breathing in it – if you are bunged up, use your mouth, it's OK!

MINDFUL CYCLE MEDITATION

Get yourself comfortable either sitting or lying down. Take a moment to take in your surroundings before you close your eyes.

Close your eyes and take five deep breaths, breathing right into your belly, and allow that breath to fully leave your body. There is no rush – just feel that breath coming into your body through your nose, and out of your body through your nose.

Let your breath return to its normal, easy rhythm. As you are breathing, allow your body to soften into whatever is supporting you. Feel the tension soften and ease, letting your body become relaxed and held. If something doesn't feel comfortable, adjust so that it is. Listen to your body as it speaks to you. This will allow you to soften and let go.

Allow your breathing to go at its normal pace – if your mind begins to wander, bring it back to the breath. Notice where you feel it: do you notice it coming into your nose, your throat, your chest or perhaps your tummy? Take a moment to notice where you feel the breath, and when you find your mind wanders as it will, bring it back to that feeling. It doesn't matter how often you need to do that: every time you notice you have wandered off, it is a mindful moment, and it is strengthening your ability to choose where you place your attention.

Imagine yourself in a beautiful garden. It is a warm, sunny day, you are surrounded by bright flowers, and the grass is lush and soft. You slip off your shoes and feel the grass between your toes, you can see a fountain in the distance, and you walk towards it.

There are five steps down to the fountain, you count them down as you take them – five, four, three, two, one. The stones are warm on your feet, and you notice that there is a comfy sun lounger that looks inviting, so you decide to lie out on it and feel the warm sun on your skin.

I invite you to place your hands on your pelvic space below your belly button. I wonder if you can take your breath all the way down to your pelvis. It doesn't matter if you can't – just enjoy the warmth and feeling of your hands on your belly.

As you lie here in the sun, feeling comfortable and at ease, can you ask yourself what it is your body really needs in this moment? Are you feeling tired? Is there tightness anywhere? Are there pleasant feelings that are subtle and distant, and could you draw them closer? Start at your head, scan across your face, eyes, jaw: do they feel relaxed or tight? Is there anything you can let go of?

Allow yourself to scan down your neck, shoulders, upper back, arms, all the way down to your hands and fingers. What are the sensations that you are feeling there? It could be something, it could be nothing at all. Just hold your curiosity to feel into the small parts of your body.

Carry on scanning down your chest, tummy, lower back, pelvis, hips and bum. What can you feel? Are there areas that feel relaxed, tight or numb? No judgements – just notice what is in your body, allow it to talk to you.

Carry on scanning down your thighs, knees, lower legs, ankles, feet and toes. What do you feel? Can you allow the muscles to soften a little more? Take a deep breath in and as you exhale, see if you can let your body sink further into the place it is being held.

Now you have scanned your body, can you notice what your body is needing? Allow yourself to take a few moments to listen to what it is saying. Do you know where you are in your cycle? What can you do today to treat your body to something wonderful? What would that look like for you?

Take a moment on your sun lounger to think about this, feeling the warmth of the sun on your body.

You have had a beautiful break in your day in this garden on the sun lounger, but you know it's time to go back to the rest of your day with the knowledge your body has given you. You climb up the steps and go back over the grass to find your shoes. You have one last look around the garden and slip though the gate and close it behind you, knowing it is always there for another time.

Start to wiggle your fingers and toes, gently moving your body and taking an easy stretch. Open your eyes when you feel ready and take a look at your surroundings. Allow yourself to come back to earth with a soft landing.

Have a drink of water after your relaxation, and I always suggest having a little journal for any thoughts or feelings that may have come up for you.

MENTAL DETOX AND CLEARING THE CLUTTER

Meditation is a form of mental detoxing, but there are other active steps we can follow to help clear the clutter when there are too many tabs open in our heads.

We need to know we have clutter to clear. Some of us are literally walking around with a hoarder's amount of baggage in our heads: the to-do lists, the jobs, the must-dos, remembering things for others, etc. Please write it down! I'm a big fan of delegation – if there is more than one person living in the house, it's down to all those people to help (unless they are under two years old, perhaps)! It's a fair point to make, though, that housework is not gendered and it belongs to everyone.

And it's not only our heads that can benefit from a regular decluttering. If our living environments start to unravel, it can be VERY cathartic to straighten that out and give it a spruce up. There is something wonderfully nurturing about clearing a space. It has been shown that our physical environments impact our brains, emotions and behaviour.[33] We are more likely to activate the 'I can't be arsed' button when things are upside down, which influences poorer choices when it comes to our coping mechanisms, such as slobbing out in front of the TV with snacks rather than do the things we need.

Ways to tackle the clutter:

- Spend 15 minutes each night before going to bed doing a quick tidy up.
- Get a cleaner – it's amazing how much tidying gets done when you have someone coming to clean the house!
- Invite friends around. This can help you get your bum in gear to tidy up, or they could also lend a hand to help you.
- Write a list of jobs for each room and work through them, even if it's just one room a week.
- Put your phone down and turn off the TV for an evening.
- Create a rota of jobs.
- Delegate!

A lot of my clients find this one tricky, so bear with. If you live with other humans, then unless they are very small, they can all have age-appropriate tasks to do. You aren't here to do everything for everyone! Asking for help isn't weak. Sharing the load of house admin is essential and personally, I feel strongly that we should be able to say, 'I have my period, I need extra help,' or 'I don't have the capacity.' If you are living with yourself, then future friending can be helpful: do all you can when you feel your best, so that during your period, you have done things that will help you beforehand. Or, reach out to friends and/or family if you need a hand.

UNDERSTANDING YOUR OWN NEEDS

When I did my nursing training, I had to study the Activities of Daily Living (ADLs) and Maslow's Hierarchy of Needs. Both of these list the things we need, as humans, to be able to survive and, in the case of Maslow's Hierarchy, thrive.

ADLs are activities we need to be able to do in order to look after ourselves. These are:

- Movement
- Nourishment
- Dressing
- Personal hygiene
- Getting to the toilet

Maslow's Hierarchy of Needs is often portrayed as a pyramid, with each set of needs building on top of each other. Physiological needs is the foundation (on the bottom at number 5) and the most fundamental, and we go up from there:

1. Self-actualisation – knowing you're the queen of fucking everything
2. Esteem – Respect, strength, self-esteem, freedom
3. Love and belonging – sense of connection with friends, family, partners, your community and environment, intimacy and sex
4. Safety – personal security, finance, a home, resources
5. Physiological – basic needs of water, food, air, shelter, sleep

In terms of our period health, all of these can be and are affected when we have issues with our menstrual cycles. I usually find my clients are on the floor when they get to me, without hope of ever thriving again. Humans are motivated by pleasure and pain – we walk towards pleasure and away from pain. When it comes to meeting our own needs, we often have no clue what they are, or even stop to consider the question! We're too caught up in the business of doing.

I FEEL THE NEED – THE NEED FOR MY NEEDS TO BE MET, ACTUALLY

But if you don't understand what your needs are, how are you going to be able to tell someone else? We feel resentment and frustration 99% of the time when we are energetically on the floor because we aren't getting our needs met – and we aren't even sure what those needs are. Often, we refuse help because we tell ourselves it's easier if we do everything on our own.

Being strong and resilient doesn't mean we never, ever ask for help – it's quite the opposite, actually. We can't just expect others to mind-read or see what needs to be done. We need to be crystal clear in our communication. That's something that doesn't always come easy, I know.

Look at the lists of ADLs and Maslow's Hierarchy, and create your own based around your menstrual needs. I invite you to really be honest with yourself about how you are caring for yourself with regards to your periods and hormones. Don't judge yourself, just write it down: where you are and where you would like to be. Then, you start to be able to see the steps you need to start taking. Make two lists one for your overall cycle and then one for your period. It might look like this...

During my cycle:

- I need to move my body every day, especially my lower back and pelvis.
- I need to have comfy clothes – no bras that dig in.
- I need regular orgasms in my life.
- I need to have a bath once a week.
- I need to use products that are as clean as possible.

- I need to make sure I drink two litres of water daily.
- I need to empty my bladder fully and not rush off the loo but wait a bit!

During my period:

- I need gentle movement during my bleed – walking only.
- I need apple crumble, dates, raw cacao and peanut butter.
- I need more sleep, and I need early nights.
- I need my period pants and reusable pads.
- I need to be able to go to the loo freely and often.

By looking at your needs like this, you can start to plan your life a little better and figure out what you need to put in place for when these needs arise. For example, I make sure I have organic cotton disposable pads when I am travelling because the fanny admin of reusables is too much at that time. Having such things in place will also enable you to add ease and joy into the mix, which is fundamental for me in all I do, even when having my period!

A lot of the time, I see clients who are frantic with tasks, have demoted themselves to the bottom of the priority list, and feel like they have to do it all and they can't. Deep down, they probably don't even want to.

I will say this again, **YOU ARE THE MOST IMPORTANT PERSON IN YOUR OWN LIFE.** Having these fundamental needs addressed and met will make you a nicer person. It might take a bit of adjustment, and you'll have to say 'NO' – yes, it is a full sentence – but it's where the magic resides.

This narrative of having it all was a total failing of the feminism department of the 90s. It just created even more pressure to do it all, in heels, backwards. We aren't meant to be everything to all people. We are, however, meant to be everything for ourselves and meant to choose our people carefully. You need to be something special to reside at my table, end of, next please.

THE SEASONS OF OUR NEEDS

When we start to put together our lists of needs with the seasons of our cycle, we can really begin to see where our needs aren't being met. When things get feral in our autumn phase, for example, it's the emotional part of our needs that isn't being met. If we are in pain or heavy or knackered, we won't want to do most of the things being asked of us – our bodies aren't at full capacity. So, we get tired, and our patience wears thin, and we get short-fused. Pair that with hormones being out of balance and our adrenals being tired, and it's the perfect storm.

Resting and cutting back is one of the best things you can actually do for yourself whenever you feel like this. Get real with how much you *want* to cope with, not *can* cope with. There is a difference, and you don't have to do everything! The exercise below will show you what drains you and what lifts you up. We need less drains and more joy, but remember: each of us is unique. And if you find this a bit hard, that's telling! Investing in yourself isn't a luxury, and it doesn't have to be fancy. Think micro and macro here; that way, there is a bigger chance of making the changes you need.

I would do one of these lists for each quarter of the month – seriously, give it a go because your needs will be different in each phase. I bet my wardrobe of sequins on it. Start putting you first, and big, spangly shizzle is gonna happen.

EXERCISE: I invite you to write down a Joy List and a Drain List. Be honest with yourself as to what lights you up and what brings you down. Where are you spending most of your time? And where might you like to spend your time?

A NOTE ON NOT-SO-SOCIAL MEDIA

It's easy to get highjacked from your own path, but comparing yourself to others is never a great idea – no good can come of it. Being swept up in the toxic productivity it often promotes will have you ping-ponging around the place like you're in a pinball machine. Have you ever stopped to ask yourself if you really want to be doing half the things you think you are supposed to be doing?

If you are noticing yourself getting cranky or jealous when you are on social media – PUT IT DOWN. You are always in control of what you are seeing. It's the same with the news – it's important to take breaks from watching it. However, it can be very comforting sometimes to watch reels of dogs doing cute things – it's why they are so popular! If you find yourself doom-scrolling and feeding that part of you that is scared/angry/bored or all three, this is a sign you need to change things up and do something wholesome away from your phone instead.

YOU ARE THE AWESOME – DON'T LET ANYONE TELL YOU OTHERWISE

I cannot tell the people I meet and work with enough how wonderful they are, how they are needed in this world to do the things they need to do, that they light up rooms, make others smile and laugh, and are so loved beyond their wildest dreams. See yourself through the eyes of those that love you.

This slippery, invisible, meta stuff is hard and unyielding in its need for commitment from us to get a handle on it, and we are mostly ill-equipped or blissfully ignorant to the job. The reward for sifting through your own shit is that you get to plant new things that will flourish in it. Remember, you are in control of this ship, and I hope this section will give you better coordinates for navigation.

DO YOU HAVE BOUNDARIES MADE OF JELLY?

It takes practise to put yourself first, for your own good and the benefit of everyone around you, and many of us struggle to put – and keep – the necessary boundaries in place to support this. If you have boundaries made of jelly, work on making them stronger. It might make your ass sweat to start with, but it's ultimately a breath of fresh air. Creating stronger boundaries can look like:

- Stopping people-pleasing
- Saying no
- Blocking or hiding people on the socials
- Removing toxic humans and/or situations from your life
- Only doing things that make you fizz
- Stopping comparing yourself to others
- Allowing yourself to fully embody your achievements and basking in that glory
- Coronating yourself as the queen of your own fucking universe
- Creating and tailoring your own top table – only those with an invite get to dine with you
- Sacking off those around you that don't have your best interests at heart, and you will know who they are – they generally show themselves by telling you, 'You've changed'

When I didn't understand the importance of myself, my power, what I am here to do in the world, my love, shared joy, dancing, sequins and ability to make people laugh – which others saw BTW! – I kept trying to hijack situations, unconsciously most of the time, and then I wondered why things were going sideways all the time. I did a lot of eye-rolling and saying, 'But you don't understand.' Then, I started investing in myself and it was a game changer. So, I get it.

If this makes you want to poke me in the eye, or makes you feel nauseous or angry, I want you to sit with that for a bit and explore it. This is your system telling you that it knows – it knows that you are hiding and would really like to break that box open, try it all on, leave what doesn't fit anymore behind, and then move on into a world of wonder, a world of you.

ADDRESSING TOXIC PRODUCTIVITY AND BURNOUT

'Toxic productivity' is a term that has its roots in the patriarchy, capitalism and systemic racism, and it's gaining traction. It's basically the concept of always living in the sun, trying to maintain unhealthy levels of perfectionism, success and goals. It's a concept that wants us to wake up, work, go to bed and repeat, until we hop off this mortal coil. No joy, no whimsy, just nose to the grindstone, because if it ain't worth the graft, then it ain't worth having!

This is like living in the daylight all the time, which, as anyone who does that will tell you, is hard because you have no off button at night. We need both activity AND rest. When you have your little rest after your yoga session, that is where all the hard work comes together! It is not weak, shameful, unhealthy, sad, fake or worthless to rest. If you do not rest, you will harm your body!

'Allostatic load' is the technical term for being well and truly wrung out and burned out; it's when your body pulls the emergency-stop button. It can feel very foggy here, like you are tired all the time, even after sleep, because you aren't resting if you get into bed and just read another chapter, or watch another episode, or talk about that issue a bit more. YOU NEED TO BE TUCKED UP IN BED! Rest is rest is rest.

Burnout happens when we dismiss all the warning signs that have come before.

A farmer is sitting on his porch in a chair, hanging out. A friend walks up to the porch to say hello, and hears an awful yelping, squealing sound coming from inside the house. 'What's that terrifyin' sound?' asks the friend.

'It's my dog,' says the farmer, 'He's sittin' on a nail.'
'Why doesn't he just get off it?' asks the friend. The farmer
deliberates on this and replies, 'Doesn't hurt enough yet.'[34]

There is waxing and waning with all of life's adventures, but if you don't make the time for you, no one else will. Even your wonderful partner, kids, family and friends won't know you need help if you never ask.

There are lots of other people
ready to tear us down,
some of them we are related to,
we don't need to be
doing it to ourselves.
  – A Gemma-ism

Get outside

Nature is an excellent antidote for burnout and toxic productivity, among plenty of other things. Sitting under an expansive sky or a big tree can and does scale our perception of our problems.

In her amazing podcast *The Three-Day Effect*, Florence Williams examines how being in nature for a minimum of three days changes up the chemicals in our bodies. It softens our stress responses, creates more of the good chemicals to float around our bodies and literally makes us feel better.[35]

Getting out in nature for just half an hour a day can make all the difference to us – in fact, even tiny bursts of time outside lift our moods – and even looking at pictures or listening to sounds of nature have been shown to produce benefits.

Being in nature increases serotonin and dopamine levels, which boosts mood and motivation. And luckily, nature is something most of us have access to; if you don't know where the nearest park or beach or common is, you might be encouraged to seek out places near you that you haven't been – yet.

AFFIRMATIONS

Affirmations are amazing – they can really put a pep in your stride. They are positive statements that encourage a positive mental attitude and help drive away self-sabotaging and negative thoughts. Think it sounds crazy? Well, we affirmate all the time but generally in a negative way. And they are felt with more pizzazz in the body when they start with 'I AM'.

Here is an invitation to play with some personal affirmations for yourself. I will kick you off, but I encourage you to write your own list. Then, put them up around the house or record yourself reciting them and listen to them back – I know, I cringe at the sound of my own voice too, but they're more powerful if you hear them coming from your own voice. This is powerful shizzle, babes.

Here are some of my favourite affirmations to inspire your list:

- I am fucking awesome.
- I am confident. I walk with swagger.
- I am more than enough.
- I am so enough. I spill out and shine bright.
- I am one hot ass biatch.
- I am a sex pot. I shoot glitter beams out my fanny.
- I am so clever. I have amazing ideas.
- I am a star-studded super queen.
- I am love. I love myself first.
- I am discerning about who is in my inner circle.

Writing these has made me laugh, and I look forward to hearing what you come up with. Please share them with me on the socials – links to my accounts on page 243 of the book!

Right, let's crack on, but whenever you need a fix of cheer, head back to this section. And remember: it's no accident you are here on this planet, you are just fucking awesome. Carry on!

CHAPTER 15 ROUND-UP

Slowing down can be a challenge – it isn't on the agenda for the patriarchal capitalist society we live in. Giving yourself the permission to stop is quite the rebellious task, though, and if I know anything about my crew, I know they like being rebels. Here are the takeaways from this chapter:

- Put your phone down. I promise the world won't end – some of us remember a time they didn't exist!
- Sit still for 30 seconds and concentrate on your breathing. Put your hand on your chest or belly to connect with it.
- GET OUTSIDE EVERY DAY!
- Record the meditation on page 190, kick back and listen to it (or listen to it on my website – see page 243 to find a link).
- Clear away physical clutter and see how different you feel in a clearer space.
- Figure out your needs during your cycle. Have an audit through the month and see what comes up for you.
- Set some boundaries for yourself.
- Use the affirmations or create your own!

CHAPTER 16

PERIOD STIGMA AND SHAME

The active ingredient in period stigma is misogyny.

Lindy West

When my period arrived, I remember saying to a friend, with some modicum of pride, that I was finally a woman. I was 14, I was laughed at, ridiculed and told not to be so stupid. Nothing was really explained to me by my mum. I was just presented with a packet of Kotex period pads, which felt like rough breeze blocks in my pants. If I picked up the pace running for the bus, they would shimmy up the back of my pants and try and make a bid for freedom over the top of my trousers. Swan-diving period pads are up there with the worst thing that could happen to you at 14. I'm pre-wings – *pre-wings*, people!!

Talking about our periods, cycles and hormones helps to normalise them for others. You know how you feel seen when you see someone that looks like you on the TV, or when you see someone doing something you want to do? It gives you a sense of 'actually, I *can* do this because they are', and it's the same thing for period health – if we start to change the culture, it benefits all of us in the long run. I'm not suggesting you have to do cartwheels through the office announcing you are going to change your tampon, but if you do, please, for the love of god, tag me in that post because it will go viral.

CHALLENGE PERIOD STIGMA

So, all that said, how can we challenge the stigma of periods and the way we think about them? Here is my six-point manifesto.

1. **Get to know your period.**
   By this I don't mean smear it all over your face and take pictures of yourself. (True story, someone did this and it ended up in the paper. If it's something you want to do then go for it.) I mean get geeky about it and chart it. When I say charting, I mean more than noting down when it starts and stops – I mean documenting every day what is occurring with your cycle. I promise you this is illuminating; you will start to find out so much more about yourself that you might not have even known was there. See Chapter 4 for more details on this.

2. **Talk to your partner about it.**
   I know that back in the day, I didn't mention anything about my period to my boyfriends, and not even to my husband, particularly. Now, he knows my cycle, and the array of paraphernalia that accompanies my periods these days offers another heads up. Steams, pads, watering plants with the water from rinsing my pads, and watching the look on people's faces when they ask why the orchids in the bathroom look amazing! (Lol – obvs, you don't have to do that, but your period blood is full of stem cells which literally make things grow, so if you have a sick house plant, try it!) I tell you, once you start talking about your period, you won't want to stop, because it's fun to challenge and watch the reactions of others. The more you do it, the more normalised if becomes, and then it' will just be how you roll. You will inspire others to do the same.

When you get conscious of the often-negative reactions that people have about a natural bodily function, it starts to become apparent that we need to talk about this so much more than we already do. Take period sex, for example. There is no right or wrong, whatever works for you; an orgasm can be helpful during your period because it contracts the uterus, and this can help relieve pain and expel any blood that might not be coming out due to a tilted pelvis.

3. **Ask for period products to be put in the toilets in your places of work.**
   It should be standard for these to be supplied, and I don't know about you, but I am fed up at the number of times I have been caught short without at pad – thanks, irregular period – only to have to make one out of loo roll, which does the exact same bid for freedom as the Kotex of my youth did. I always ask in cafés if they could please put a basket of period products in the bathroom. It might not happen straight away, but if enough people ask for it, change will come.

4. **Stop hiding your period product up your sleeve.**
   You don't need to do this. You have nothing to be ashamed of, and I would really ask why you feel the need to do this (if you do), and there will be some work to be done, for sure. It might be weird the first few times you go to the bathroom with your pad or tampon in your hand, but I promise you, people seeing it won't freak out. In fact, more often than not when I ask people to do this, they report back that either no one batted an eyelid, or a conversation happened that was beneficial to all.

   I also want to add here that you might feel that everyone is looking at you, but they aren't really. Coming from someone who has died on her ass in front of an audience a few times, where everyone really was looking at me, humans forget stuff really quickly. Pete won't be going down the pub saying, 'Oh my god, Fiona was holding a tampon in her hand on the way to the bathroom today and I saw it, I must leave.' We are so caught up in our own thoughts and situations, we really don't see much of what is going on. Put yourself in both scenarios and explore how you might think. If you have judgements about this, what is that telling you? Challenge yourself, because chances are, they aren't your stories you are telling yourself, they are stories that were given to you, and you know what? You can change those anytime you like.

5. **Have conversations with your children.**
Support them, allow them to ask questions and learn together. If you are particularly good at talking about periods (it might surprise you to know that I have been lined up to give the period chat to quite a few children of my friends and family!), then help out where you can with 'the talk'. Make it fun, engaging and informative – all the things you probably never had. There are books about it to help, and you make a little celebration of it when the first one arrives – doesn't have to be anything fancy, although chocolate cake is always a winner. Just don't ignore it or laugh and joke about it, making the person feel small. That shit stays with people.

6. **Speak the words that are our biology.**
Euphemisms will always be part of our culture with periods, and they have been around a long time, but they don't help when you are trying to change the narrative with yourself and others. Calling it 'that time of the month' or 'shark week' doesn't help anyone. Using the word 'period' or 'menstruation' shouldn't make people cringe.

The fact it does means we need to use it all the more until it's as functional as saying 'shoe'. Same goes for body parts – telling your child they have a 'foof' or 'lady garden' is pretty confusing. Actually, these words can be a good way of breaking down tensions when you start talking to teens about all of this. You can list together all the ridiculous names that are used, but then talk about the proper names – no one wants to be the person that puts their hand up in sex ed class and says, 'It's called a nooni.' School is hard enough, people.

So, I am saying, stop hiding your tampon up your sleeve to go to the toilet. Have a selection of period products in your toilets, and have a conversation about the fact you might need to work from home when you have your period because it feels like the earth is falling from your legs. It will feel cringy to start because you are stepping out of a norm, but I can't do this on my own, I'm a drop in the ocean, and I need you all behind me waving your tampons like you don't care.

This is about having conversations with your partners, your kids – especially the men in your family. It's owning the fact you bleed, or you are going through the perimenopause, or that you are tired from all the bleeding, or you are in pain and can't be at full capacity because you are bleeding.

Seriously, if this were a condition of the penis, we wouldn't stop hearing about it and seeing adverts that it's OK to ask for penis period leave. There would be care in place, there would be research. The only way we will get change is by being the change, and that means taking one for the team and speaking up. Even when you feel on your own, you know you have the collective behind you. We owe it to ourselves and those behind us to make a difference with this bleedy narrative that is at best archaic, but worse still, damaging our chances to live normal, stigma-free lives.

A LONG WAY TO GO

Around the world, getting your period can mean many different things. Sat in your home, a café, wherever you are reading this, it can feel that optimum period health care is a million miles away from being the norm – and I have been moaning my ass off a lot about that! We are, however, living like queens in comparison to other women and girls around the globe. I want you to know that every time you stand up for or challenge something, you are changing the collective not just around you, but around the world. Shining a light on what others must endure can be hard to take on, but it's important to know our privilege and use that to help as a collective for others – we are all in this together after, all.

In some parts of the world, periods are thought to make the woman experiencing them dirty and unclean. They are ostracised from their communities in sometimes dangerous and unsanitary environments. If you live in a place where it is deeply shameful to talk openly about menstruation, even in an educational capacity, how the hell is anyone meant to get to the actual facts of things?! Deepening our understanding of this and our own privilege around this is important. But there is work to do everywhere. Even in developed nations, period poverty is a real deal, and there is a big movement to make this not be the case.

It is estimated that around 137,000 girls in the UK miss school each year because of a lack of access to period products. There are also reports of girls having to use socks or the same pad all day[36] – loo roll isn't a period product, by the way. Periods are horrific for women who are homeless – have you ever stopped to think of that nightmare? When period products started to appear in public toilets, some people were bemoaning the fact they might get stolen. Well, yes, they might, but probably by someone who needs them. You can get condoms for free; sex is a choice, but a period is not.

We paid 5% luxury tax on all our period products in the UK for years. I just can't get my head around that; however, at the time of writing this book, this has recently been abolished.[37] Moreover, in Scotland, free period products are available to all and are in schools, colleges and hospitals. In much of the rest of the UK, however, it is still very hit-or-miss as to whether or not we have access to free period products. Given that they are expensive, we are all very generous in helping each other out if we get caught short.

That's why, as I said before, talking about our periods is so important. Remember the collective gasp when the Olympic swimmer Fu Yuanhui announced she didn't do so well because she had her period? It was in the news for a week! She was bent double with cramps and broke the 'taboo' of mentioning she had her period – in 2016! Because of her comments, she became a national hero for many women, especially in China, where period education isn't as progressive.[38] British sprinter Dina Asher-Smith was also praised for mentioning she had her period and that it affected her performance during the competition.[39] Those using their platforms to raise awareness and open up a conversation are true champions.

Talking about our periods helps to break down myths, like using tampons will mean you aren't a virgin. Virginity is a whole load of patriarchal BS in and of itself. Losing your virginity as a male is celebrated, whereas for women, it is seen as the most heinous crime against your virtue. I mean, I didn't lose my virginity – I knew exactly where I put it!

So, be brave, make it easier for those coming after and, where you can, take an activist/advocate role for women in parts of the world that are way behind on this.

Sometimes it can feel cringy and uncomfortable to speak up about periods, but know that every time you do, it does make a difference. You are paving the way for those that follow. Plus, I can't do all this on my own – I need my period groupies to go forth and spread the message. You can do this to your capacity. You don't have to be the same as me or the next person, but the very fact that you take the torch and run with it means we are all singing from the same song sheet.

CHAPTER 16 ROUND-UP

Remember: there is nothing to be ashamed about with having a period or feeling the effects of hormones. Say those exact words; no one can argue with you, because 'tis the truth!

We have reached the end of Part 2 – woohoo! I hope you have gained some deeper insights into yourself and your body. Cultivating some agency over ourselves is so deliciously against the system, you total rebellious legends!

It's a lot to take in, I know. I wouldn't be surprised if you feel a range of emotions. I know I did when I started doing this work, and it's all perfectly OK.

My hope it you now realise you have way more scope to change things up than what you may have been led to believe.

PART 3

HEADING INTO MENOPAUSE

Women are like teabags. We don't know our true strength until we are in hot water.

Eleanor Roosevelt

I wanted to acknowledge the ending bit to our hormones. This book is about periods and hormonal health, but everything in it – how to care for yourself and your hormones – applies to this window too. Everything you do now is paying into your hormonal pension pot, as it were.

For some of us, we long to see the back of our periods; for others it's a bittersweet goodbye. I would say for the vast majority, it's like stumbling alone in the dark, bumping our shins into the sharp corners of night sweats and dry vaginas that we had absolutely no bloody idea to expect.

Welcome to the whole new world of the perimenopause and menopause. To get all Elton John and sing 'Circle of Life' at you, this is another bit of that cycle, but you don't have periods anymore. You can strike that bit of fanny admin off your list for good. Hurrah!

You will have a bit of a scenic route to get there, though – a sort of reverse puberty, with hair growing in new places like chins and boobs. Meno doesn't happen overnight, unlike the chin hairs, so here's a bit of info about what happens next...

Dun dun dunnnn!

CHAPTER 17

THE PERIMENOPAUSE: WELCOME TO LIMBO LAND

The moment in between what you once were, and who you are now becoming, is where the dance of life really takes place.

Barbara De Angelis

The perimenopause seems to confuse the hell out of everyone. I mean, as we have learnt thus far, it's hardly surprising, given so much about our bodies has been written out, overlooked or derailed over the course of time. However, this is a part of our period career that has been given even less airtime – until recently.

I want to say that a chapter on this is by no means enough – I could write a whole book just about the perimenopause. There is a lot going on, but it doesn't have to be the car crash it's billed to be, either. Again, it's about finding your body literacy, because we are on shifting sands during this time of life, in more than one department.

We generally start to notice perimenopausal symptoms in our 40s, but it actually starts in our late 30s. It can feel a bit bleak, like we are falling off the radar, when actually it's a new chapter and lease of life. I absolutely HATE the narrative that turning 40 is a bad thing – getting older is a privilege not afforded to everyone!

Yes, with it comes not being able to get up out of a chair without making a noise, but it also brings a wealth of riches. Please don't play into the hands of the narrative that women are only useful youthful – that belongs in the dark ages. You are needed at every stage of your life. We ALL have something to offer and a light to shine, and I won't be swayed on that.

WHAT IS THE PERIMENOPAUSE?

The perimenopause is the time when you still have cycles but they start to show signs and symptoms of the menopause, which is when they stop. The perimenopause can last as long as 15 years, but the average is around 4 years – although the average really doesn't tell us anything (I'll say more on this later).

The first sign that we tend to notice is a change in cycle length – they usually get shorter. If, like me, you have had an irregular cycle, and then get it regular just in time for it all to go out the window again – I FEEL you. Those that have always had an irregular cycle will be used to this, but those that have been regular as clockwork, a bit of advice: just don't bother with white pants for a few years, OK?!

If we take the analogy of the seasons of the cycle, we can use the same structure for the seasons of our period careers:

- Spring = puberty
- Summer = the main part of our period career
- Autumn = perimenopause
- Winter = menopause/post menopause

Perimenopause is like puberty in reverse, if you can remember what that was like! It was pretty erratic, having strange periods with no regularity. Nothing was ever quite even until you were a couple years into having those hormones coursing through your body. When you think about it, it's a lot to take on board at a young age, to be honest!

As we enter our peri years, our bodies are winding down from their period careers; the parts responsible for periods start handing over to other parts of our endocrine systems and getting ready for retirement. It can seem a bit bleak but there is a new lease of life after all of this. I feel strongly that it should get a better PR campaign because it really doesn't have to be a shitshow.

The changes can be subtle at first, and for some it can build up to be a bit of a rollercoaster ride. Some can walk this stage without too many symptoms; others will be somewhere in between.

WHAT HAPPENS?

It isn't as simple as our oestrogen just dropping, and it isn't because we run out of eggs, either – that is a false narrative. Like all aspects of our hormones, it's complex and there are, as ever, a lot of ifs, buts and maybes to this transition.

During the perimenopause, we start to get more anovulatory cycles (where we don't ovulate) and have longer follicular phases compared to the periods we would have had in our 20s. This means that we don't get the progesterone and, therefore, there is nothing to counter the oestrogen in our bodies. Although the oestrogen is on a downward trajectory, it is the missing progesterone that we start to notice the most.

Even though perimenopause is starting to be recognised more, we are still at risk of over-simplifying it and trying to put everyone into the same box. We seem to want to create a tick-box of 'oh I'm 42 now, I must be perimenopausal, and I will stop my periods in five years' time', but it just doesn't work like that. If we start treating everyone as individuals and listening to their experiences of what is happening in their bodies, instead of trying to fit into arbitrary rules, we would be able to start doing the things we need way before we need them.

This might start helping us head into our peri and meno years in a much more positive way.

HOW LONG DOES IT LAST?

The question I get asked most often is how long will it last – a better question might be how long is a piece of string! It depends on so many factors: genetics, lifestyle, overall health, diet – we might as well put shoe sizes in there too. Roughly speaking, it kicks off before we have even heard of it in our late 30s, gathers pace in our 40s and might be done by our 50s or even 60s, depending on when it starts, in that vague lots-of-numbers way. If you have learnt nothing else by the end of this book, I hope you at least realise that working with hormones can range from varied and mysterious, to clockwork and predictive, and it is hugely personal to every single one of us.

WHAT ARE THE SYMPTOMS?

There are simply gazillions of symptoms for the perimenopause, but here are some of the more common ones:

- Changes to the flow of your period – heavy, lighter, shorter, longer, etc.
- Cycle-length changes – longer or shorter or a combination of both
- Increased PMS
- Fatigue
- Sleep disruptions
- Raging at everything, everyone, all the time
- Brain fog
- A fuzzy memory
- Sore boobs
- Headaches and migraines
- The bloats
- Hot flushes

- Night sweats
- Dry eyes/mouth
- Joint and muscle pain
- Vaginal dryness
- Changes to libido, from not bothered to can't get enough
- Discomfort with penetrative sex
- Panic attacks
- Mood changes, such as anxiety and depression
- Changes to skin – dryness, acne, oiliness, loss of elasticity, etc.
- Itchy skin
- Hair thinning or loss (also check thyroid levels if this happens)
- Diarrhoea and/or constipation

I mean, who's in?! Sign me up, right? I'm sorry that list will have sucked all the good humour out of the room, but it is important that you know, so you can help yourself and advocate for yourself about what *you* are experiencing. Otherwise, you can be forgiven for thinking you are going a little bit crazy.

The other day I completely lost the word 'milk' from my brain. I had to explain to the bemused young lad behind the counter I wanted the white stuff in my tea, but not from cows, from coconuts! We got there in the end. It's normal for this to happen; it's new to me but I am embracing it. It gives me a whole load of material to use on stage if nothing else.

I know it can feel a bit terrifying that these changes are afoot, but forewarned is forearmed, and I believe we can get through the shittiest of times with knowledge (and a bit of a sense of humour).

It's really important to get to know your own personal landscape at this time. As with menstrual health, we all kinda do it the same, but then we also don't at all – there are lots of personal idiosyncrasies. The perimenopause is no different: it will be your own personal journey but thinking about it before it happens, or starting to get a handle of it if you are already there, is going to be beneficial to you. I hope by now you are realising that this stuff we are learning about ourselves is never wasted.

TO HRT, OR NOT TO HRT? THAT IS THE QUESTION

I don't want to throw anyone shade here for their choices – both are valid as long as you have gone in with your eyes open. I will say, though, you don't have to do the menopause with HRT (hormone replacement therapy). This stage in life isn't a disease that needs to be treated; it is a natural process of your existence.

There will be those of you that don't want to take HRT, can't take it, or take it and don't get on with it, and the danger of the 'this is the only way you should do it' narrative is that it alienates those that fall outside of the HRT range.

The perimenopause can stick a spanner in the works for sure, and that might have you running for the drugs. BUT you actually want *less* oestrogen in the lead-up to menopause because your body needs to become used to running on less of the stuff. This will make for a smoother entry to menopause when those levels inevitably drop.

If you have an early menopause (whereby all your periods have ceased before the age of 40), or you have a full hysterectomy with removal of ovaries before you are in the place to go through the menopause, then HRT is a sensible and much-needed option for you. You need your hormones, and having them removed abruptly, or stopping before they should, is less than ideal – I will talk more on this in the menopause chapter.

I work with many clients to help them find their feet through this transition. It's important to keep your own hormones flying for as long as possible so that you get all the goodies from them, which further supports my argument that all of this is less about making babies and more about making hormones to keep us healthy.

WHERE DO YOU SIT WITH YOUR MIDLIFE AWAKENING?

I vote we cancel calling it a 'midlife crisis' – the definition of crisis in the dictionary is 'a time of intense difficulty or danger.' Midlife it isn't a crisis, FFS, it's a new stage of life where we get to take stock and adjust accordingly. That is not a crisis – that is a transition. Calling it a crisis implies we have no control over it, whereas calling it a transition keeps us in the driving seat.

We definitely have this narrative that it is the end of the world, that we are heading down a path we can't help, and we are on the perimenopause roller coaster whether we want to be or not. The thing is, though, not all women have symptoms. Sure, there will be some that we know, but in some places around the world, the transition isn't as marked, or there are not words for it in the language, which I think is always telling!

Again, the studies on this are a little sparse, but without doubt, our fast-paced lives in the West have a massive influence on how we perceive our changing bodies. Basically, all the points that I have touched on throughout the course of this book concerning the health of our periods, cycles and hormones are just as important during perimenopause and menopause. It is a life's work, of which we were never made to understand the real importance. Postmenopausal life is a complex social and cross-cultural conundrum. Declining oestrogen is just one of the numerous pieces that make up the puzzle.

There is also the impact of how we use our bodies in the West to birth humanity, and it looks very different to other cultures around the globe, where women often have less personal choice. We might not ever be pregnant, or we might only have a couple of pregnancies. We might not breastfeed, or we might do it for a couple weeks or months or years. We might pop out babies earlier or later in our lives. It all causes change and impacts us. This is not to say we should be barefoot and pregnant our entire lives, but the hormone soup in which we percolate our bodies during these experiences will change the playing field!

For example, using synthetic hormones ages the cervix because it makes it work harder to produce its thick secretions. We would normally create this secretion at our infertile points in our cycle only, not all the time. So, considering that I was on the pill for ten years, my cervix is ten years older because of that. If I had had a child, however, it would have repaired that ageing process. I've made peace with the fact I have a 52-year-old cervix at the age of 42, and knowing that doesn't make me want to change the choices I have made. However, it does show the power of your hormones when they are growing humanity, which I think is kinda cool.

I'd also like to give a special mention to the environmental toxins we are exposed to throughout our lives, and the impact they've had, the full extent of which we may never actually know. Reducing your exposure to them will not just serve your period health but your overall health, so it is never too late to make changes on that front. There are so many products that we know to be endocrine disrupters that we will have been literally bathing in (see page 136). It just makes me think of *Erin Brockovich* every time, and I don't think that is a bad thing. Be more Erin about your products: have some agency and discernment about what you put in and on your amazing body, but also don't get paranoid, either. ☺

So, what I am trying to say, as I have maintained the whole way through this book, is that you can figure out the best route for you, and it doesn't have to be the way everyone else is going. It isn't a new thing that is happening to you, but it will be new to you, and educating yourself about it is always the best way to go.

Diet and lifestyle play a role here, too. Remember when you didn't get hangovers in your 20s and now they're three-dayers every time? Well, your body has changed, and it can't act like a 20-year-old anymore because it isn't one! There will be things that will aggravate symptoms such as hot flushes, for example – alcohol is one of the biggies here – but the detective work will come from you.

I know there will also be people out there saying it doesn't affect them, and that is where balance comes in. Personally, I gave up drinking three years ago because it just didn't suit my body anymore. I felt awful after a glass of wine, and I thought to myself, 'Is this really worth it?' For me, no, but you must find you in all this and follow what suits you. Always be curious about the causes and effects of things that will be occurring in your body.

The nutrition chapter of this book will put you in good stead for working with peri symptoms. However, if you are finding that a coffee or a glass of wine gives you an incredible hot flush, you are already learning about the landscape of your perimenopause.

I really enjoy working with perimenopause because it is sometimes the first time my clients really get to start looking after themselves, and the transformations are glorious. We can change our directions, narratives and dreams in the blink of an eye. It's all there for the taking – just sometimes we have forgotten about how bloody spectacular we are. We can still knock it out the park while having a power surge, and owning our stories is always a massively important part of the process.

SOME PRACTICAL TIPS

As you become aware that you might be in the perimenopause part of your life, there are some common symptoms that may be affecting you. Here are my top tips for supporting yourself while you navigate this new part of your journey.

CHANGES TO THE FLOW OF YOUR PERIOD AND CYCLE LENGTH

It is very worthwhile looking to support your hormones through this transition. Working through the chapters in Part 2 are where you can make the most impact for yourself. My biggest piece of advice is plan for your peri – don't wait for it to arrive and wallop you around the head. As with all hormonal issues, the normalisation of them being terrible is very real. Look where that has led us: to a place where we're struggling with feral hormones and being medicated. The peri and meno are no exception. Helping your body rid itself of inflammation, working on your gut, tweaking your diet, sleeping well, shaking your ass as often as you can and addressing stressors – ALL OF THIS is forward planning for your peri and meno pension pot.

My potions of choice for the peri are:

- Joany Crony Blend, which is specifically made for the common perimenopausal symptoms
- Bloody Brilliant Tonic, which helps to balance out hormones and iron out any kinks
- Fuck that Shit, which helps to support your nervous system and adrenals, as they can take a bit of a hit at this time

FATIGUE AND SLEEP DISRUPTIONS

These kinds of symptoms can make everything look a lot uglier. Our reserves become depleted quickly and things can start to unravel. Here are some tips for making sleep easier during the peri:

- If it's because of hot flushes and night sweats, simple actions like cooling the room down and sleeping in cotton clothing can make all the difference.
- Allow yourself some nano-naps during the day where you can, as a micro-sleep of 20 minutes max really can do wonders.
- Have a 'no phones in the bedroom' rule to allow yourself some proper time to unwind.
- Give yourself a time limit of lying in bed trying to sleep. After half an hour of trying to settle, get up, make a cuppa, read a few pages and try again. Usually, this works to help reset the body.

INCREASED PMS, THE RAGES AND MOOD CHANGES, ANXIETY AND DEPRESSION

Working with balancing your hormones can make a big difference to this part of the peri landscape. I suggest you:

- Be honest with people about where you are and about being in your perimenopause. You might do that in a joking way or in a more heartfelt manner; either way, better communication really helps everyone.
- Note any changes and assess if there are patterns. Look at external stressors or situations that can exacerbate these feelings.
- Seek help in supporting yourself through this transition. If you are struggling with your mental health, don't let that fester. This part of your life is the autumn phase, and like the autumn of your menstrual cycle, unresolved stuff will just keep knocking on your door if you ignore it.

BRAIN FOG AND FUZZY MEMORY

Your brain is rewiring again – the same happens when you start your period and are pregnant. The brain and ovaries are very much linked together. Because your hormone call centre is in the brain, there is a change in communication services as hormone levels shift, and the brain has to accommodate for that. Losing the ability to use verbs (it's not actually a scientific thing, just something I've noticed!) is pretty common. It's important you don't put pressure on yourself – this makes matters far worse. I use humour to get me through the worst of it if it happens!

- If you need to write things down more to help yourself, do it! Please embrace whatever you need to make life easier. You aren't losing your marbles; new mums go through a similar brain change, and they come out the other side!
- Be honest about it to others – don't try to hide it or feel embarrassed. If you mention it, someone else will tell you they are in the same boat.
- If you need to, become a big fan of lists, like me!

HOT FLUSHES AND NIGHT SWEATS

These can feel full on when they happen. Again, helping to balance out your hormones can make a big difference. Oestrogen on the perimenopause rollercoaster is the perpetrator.

- Food and nutrition can be triggers for this. I have mentioned about hot drinks and alcohol – you might find these aren't tolerable to you during this part of your life.
- Sleeping while wearing more natural fibres, such as cotton and linen, is very helpful. Make the most of the fact you won't need the heating on as much in the winter because you will be running hotter!
- Your liver generates a lot of heat, and it does a lot of fancy-pants cleaning during the night. Allow your liver to be working optimally by supporting it with herbs such as milk thistle (which is in my I'm Bloody Livid potion). Reducing sugars can help take off the load, as sugar is one

of the main causes of fatty liver. If bad habits have crept in, this is your opportunity to address them.

VAGINAL DRYNESS AND CHANGES TO LIBIDO

This is a big deal. Sex and everything about it is a core need. Addressing stress is a key factor in this area – if you are thinking and have too much in your head, you aren't dropping into the space. You need to be fully present with your body.

- Slowing things right down so your body has time to adjust and adapt to the feelings is really important. There is no shame in needing to have more time spent around sex.
- Lubrication can go some way to helping with vaginal dryness. Love Your Labia lip balm is my blend – it's natural, so no nasties in your nethers. I believe that if I'm not happy to eat it, I'm probably not going to want to put it on my vulva.
- Hormones can play a part in libido but, to be honest, the biggest inhibitor is stress. Feeling wired just doesn't press the passion button.
- If penetrative sex has become uncomfortable, it's worth trying lube to see if that makes a difference. Otherwise, get yourself checked out to make sure there aren't any other problems that could be causing issues.

CHAPTER 17 ROUND-UP

The perimenopause can feel like uncharted waters, mainly because it's been shrouded in mystery for most of our lifetimes. The lid is being lifted on it, thank goodness, and we are becoming more aware of this time in our lives. My advice is, don't put off making the effort to help yourself now by supporting your hormones using the information in this book. I know it feels years away for some of you, but all the work you are doing now will help with the menopause pension fund.

Working with your hormones is a long game, and we are technically always a few steps behind in it. So, making your investment to it now will pay dividends when you get there. This is the care we needed to know about from the get-go. If we were educated in hormone health, it might not seem like such a chore now to address it. Even with all my conditions, I have never looked back from working with my period and hormones, and this work has been the greatest teacher.

I would say that charting your symptoms is going to be very helpful to you during this time of our period career. It may help you to start to notice any peri symptoms and if things you are doing externally are having an impact on them. And I can't stress enough that now is the time to really start to put the elements of this book into practice to future-friend yourself going into the retirement of your period career. Please remember, however, the perimenopause is a transitional phase that won't last forever. Equally, don't ever struggle with dealing with its fallout on your own – there is plenty of help out there.

CHAPTER 18

MENOPAUSE: THE CLOAK OF INVISIBILITY SEQUINS

Men don't age better than women, they're just allowed to age.

Carrie Fisher

The menopause is a place some of us can't wait to get to – no more fanny admin, right? Wrong! There may not be any more periods, but there can still be plenty of admin to deal with. It's another time of transition, that's for sure – one I haven't gone through myself so I'm not being flippant here – but it is a time of a second wind. We are left in a place that society would have us believe is fit only for the scrap heap. We would be an asset to MI5 because we seem to become invisible to the outside world – I want to see James Bond as a gaggle of 50-somethings, no one would suspect a thing. But really, it's a time when we can find ourselves again, get reacquainted with who we were before we took on the many life roles we have gained and blend it all with who we have become.

I absolutely don't buy into the idea that we drop off the abyss like lemmings as we age, but youth is something we often try to cling to so hard that it gives us rope burns! I believe youth to be a concept rather than an aesthetic myself. However, I would be lying if I said I don't look into the brutally honest bathroom mirror of mine and see the grey hairs and laughter lines and sigh a little bit, because I've been brought up under the patriarchy along with everyone else.

But I know all about these appalling sneaky concepts now – the ones that try to pitch us against each other – and I'm not playing anymore. Don't get mad, get mischievous, and start peeling back the layers to become the you-est you there is. If that means dyeing your hair green, cutting it into a mohawk and, when you can summon up the bravery, getting your nose pierced, go bloody do it.

Ageing is a privilege. Working with kids with terminal illnesses gave me the best education there ever was – don't waste a second of this precious gift called life by trying to fit into that dress that's too small or adhering to the patriarchy's unfair standards. The second wind of menopause is just that – grab it by the partially grey pubes and run with it, babes!

WHAT IS THE MENOPAUSE?

The menopause is defined as the absence of periods for 12 months. It is the end point of the perimenopause, the phase of your menstrual hormones winding down until they stop.

- **Perimenopause** is the pre-menopause phase, lasting 4–15 years.
- **Menopause** is technically just a one-day event, as it marks the day you haven't had a period in the last 12 months.
- **Post-menopause** is where you live out the rest of your days.

It's annoying that the word 'menopause' is used to describe all three events, and I think that is very confusing for everyone.

There is a window that I mentioned in Chapter 13 between the end of your peri and the start of your post-menopause that is kind of pivotal regarding your health going forwards. It's the last two years of your peri and the first two years of your meno. It's difficult to pinpoint exactly when this is, but take note of when your periods are becoming fewer and farther between, and that is an indicator that you are there-ish.

This four-year window is where you can take all the aspects of this book and really start to tailor them to your needs. Of course, there are some changes that happen during menopause that require addressing specifically because your hormones are doing something that you are aware of – for once! Recognising the specific symptoms of falling hormones is something that can be managed with great effect with herbs, diet, lifestyle tweaks and taking stock of your mental health and well-being.

HOW LONG DOES IT TAKE?

It's difficult to know you are in the last year of your peri until it happens. You could think you are there and be 11 months in, and then you have a period and need to reset the clock back to zero and start the count again.

But once you have been period-free for 12 months, and provided you don't have any further bleeding, your menopause has been achieved. Yay!

You will not be fertile after you have gone through menopause. However, you are up until this point, so thinking about contraception is still needed, even if your periods are sometimes missing in action. It isn't unheard of to have a surprise pregnancy at this time!

WHEN WILL IT HAPPEN?

We know the answer by now, don't we… it depends! According to the *Menopause and Me* website, it usually occurs between the ages of 45–55, with the average age being 51 in the UK.[40] A mix of genetics, lifestyle and health plays a part in this as well. So, if you can find out when your mum/aunts/sisters went through theirs, it will give you a bit more of a hint for yourself.

It can seem like the best thing in the world to stop having periods early, but that can be a bit of a disaster for the health of your body. A client of mine with undiagnosed PCOS came to me because her doctor had said, 'Well, it's a bonus, isn't it, that you aren't having periods?' As I have said before, your periods are there as a report card for your health – if they aren't there when they should be, that is a red flag!

PREMATURE MENOPAUSE
There are three conditions whereby you are considered to have gone through the menopause prematurely.

- If you stop having periods before the age of 45, this is known as premature menopause.
- If your periods stop altogether before the age of 40, this is known as premature ovarian failure (POF).
- If you have a full hysterectomy (uterus and ovaries), it would put you into the menopause overnight. This would be a great shock to the system, as it is meant to be a gradual process.

All three of these conditions would ideally need to be treated with HRT (hormone replacement therapy) because you need those hormones to carry on until the time you would naturally go through the menopause. However, a surgical menopause can sometimes be required because of cancer of the uterus, breast, ovaries, etc. In that case, it might be medically advised that you don't take HRT. There is a consensus amongst experts that, where possible, ovaries should be left in place so that you have access to your hormones. If your ovaries have been removed and you can't take HRT, supporting your adrenals, gut and pancreas are very important, as are weight-bearing exercises.

WHAT ARE THE SYMPTOMS OF MENOPAUSE?

Some of the symptoms you may have experienced during peri might ramp up or ramp down, and you may have no symptoms at all, but these are some of the more common ones:

- Hot flushes
- Night sweats
- Insomnia
- Vaginal dryness
- Changes in libido, up or down
- Anxiety/depression
- Mood changes
- Rage-y ragerson
- Brain fog
- Memory short circuits

According to *Menopause and Me*, 8 out of 10 women experience some symptom of the menopause.[41] The symptoms themselves typically last around seven years after the last period.

SOME PRACTICAL TIPS

Being upfront and open about it to all the important people in your life is a very good place to start. I hope this book will have had you flexing that muscle, so by the time you are here in this chapter, you are well-versed at owning your period/hormonal situation. As well as this, it is worth taking a look at the holy trinity of lifestyle, diet and exercise, as we have in previous chapters.

LIFESTYLE

Stress is not welcome at the table at any point in time, really, but it is sometimes unavoidable. The aim should be for it to be a transient visitor, not one that stays uninvited, eating all the good snacks in the house. In middle age, when most people go through the menopause, there are several life events that can and do crop up to throw you curveballs. These might include ageing parents, children leaving home/moving away, significant people in your life becoming ill/dying, facing getting older and having breakdowns in relationships, to name but a few.

I cannot stress enough the importance of having a best practice to follow when times are tough, so you don't lose yourself to these situations entirely. Chapter 14 is relevant to all aspects of your period career, and setting yourself up to have a practice you can lean on when times are hard is going to pay dividends to you in the future.

The only thing you have any control over is yourself, how you navigate things and what you need to stay sane in challenging situations. Focusing on yourself and your boundaries is imperative. It isn't selfish to put yourself first – it's vital. Only if you are strong and grounded do you have a hope in hell of navigating the rest of it.

Herbal supplements are a wonderful way to support your system during this time. My combination of choice for my clients at this point in their period careers would be this:

- **Bloody Brilliant Tonic** – This helps with the overall balance of your hormones as they change and shift.
- **Ain't No Dried-up Prune** – This is a potion I have made specifically for the menopause. It contains a selection of herbs that are all designed to help with the common symptoms of the menopause, such as hot flushes, mood changes, brain fog, night sweats, etc.
- **Fuck that Shit** – This combination of herbs is absolutely kick-ass at helping with the anxiety, adrenal fatigue and

mood changes that can happen with hormonal shifts. It is something that can be taken every day to help conquer a stressful moment, or you can take it as and when things pop up, and you need to have a little extra support.

I am also a big advocate of taking magnesium and zinc supplements too. They are so important for our overall health, but they're two key players when it comes to hormonal health in particular.

DIET
This can play a part in how your symptoms show up. For example, alcohol does seem to make hot flushes/night sweats much worse for some. The research isn't conclusive, but it does stand to reason that during this window, you would want your liver to be in tip-top condition to help process toxins out of the body. Booze also dilates the blood vessels and can trigger a hot flush. Do your own homework on this and see if you can work out what sets things off for you.

EXERCISE
Being active in later life is important to help your body maintain fitness, but also suppleness and mobility. Weight training is a superb way to help strengthen bones and build muscle. You don't need to be built like Arnold Schwarzenegger to feel the benefits of this. Moving your body is beneficial to your overall health; being a sloth is only good for sloths.

SOME SCARY-SOUNDING CONDITIONS THAT LEAVE US FEELING WORRIED

Instead of having a blanket acceptance that all women should take HRT to sort all this out, I suggest that women would be better served by having regular check-ups on their health as a whole during this phase in life. Three of the big and scary conditions many of us may worry about at the menopause and post-menopause times of our life are osteoporosis, dementia and heart disease. Let's take a closer look.

OSTEOPOROSIS

Oestrogen is good for our bones, so as we age and our oestrogen levels lower, we do have to think seriously about our bone health. Studies have shown that early detection of bone loss is helpful,[42] but that it is more prevalent in those who have a low body mass index, prior fractures, avoided exercise,[43] given birth[44] or gone through premature menopause.[45] Taking vitamin D is helpful, as is eating a diet that is rich in calcium.

It's also important *how* we exercise, and this changes as we age. In terms of bone health, we are wanting to maintain muscle health which, in turn, helps with our bone health – it's all connected. If you are having problems in your back or neck, then it makes complete sense to work on those areas and build strength around them which, in turn, will help with bone regeneration. As with all the options that don't involve taking medication, it tends to be a scenic route – it takes commitment from you to turn up and do the thing that will make the difference you want to see. If the medications are needed after that, they will still be there.

DEMENTIA

There is a lot flying around about menopause and neurological conditions but, of course, it isn't as simple as saying that a drop in oestrogen levels causes dementia. There are links being made to our exposure to oestrogen in our lifetimes, genetics and the changes that happen in how we process oestrogen. The studies and research are assessing the *risk* of development of any and all of these conditions,[46] and I think it's important to note how stats can get skewed.

Menopause is an area of interest because women have a higher incidence of dementia than men, but more research needs to be done. The role of HRT in reducing the risk of dementia has not been confirmed, according to the British Menopause Society.[47]

Exercise is one of the top things you can do for your brain health – higher levels of exercise and physical activity combined with natural light and a healthy diet actively help to lower the chances of developing the condition in the first place. Regular activity actually increases the amount of white and grey matter in your bones – if done consecutively for a 12-week period, exercise has been found to create increased protection for the brain by lowering the levels of plaque, and increasing blood flow and cognitive functions.[48]

HEART DISEASE

The British Heart Foundation states that those who don't take HRT aren't at any more risk of having a heart attack than those that do take it.[49] There are many factors to be taken into consideration with heart disease – family history, smoking, alcohol use, exercise, diet and lifestyle, among other things.

It's going to be interesting to see where the research will go with the menopause and our health outcomes. My own opinion is that we should question everything. I am a woman who can't take HRT even if she wanted to. I understand how fearmongering and attention-grabbing these kinds of headlines can be. Fear is never a place to make sound choices from.

As with all things, it always comes down to you and what works for you. I feel that synthetic hormones have their place, but it is too arbitrary to say to all women that they must take them or else they are doomed – that just doesn't ring true to me. The global menopause market size was valued at USD $16.9 billion in 2022.[50] I think I will leave it there.

MENOPAUSE AND A CAREER

Finally, I think it is worth saying that women now make up a large portion of the workforce and, along with period conversations, menopause ones need to take place. Otherwise, we run the risk of pushing a whole swathe of experience out the door. Up to one-third of women can experience symptoms in varying degrees during the menopause that can significantly impact their quality of life. Due to the taboo nature of a perfectly normal part of the endocrine system, however, women often report greater difficulty in managing symptoms, especially at work. They feel embarrassment and fear in disclosing their status because they may be stigmatised for being menopausal.[51]

For a lot of us, having struggled through our lives and careers with our periods, we cannot suffer the same fate when it comes to the menopause. The thing that underpins all of this is the taboo nature of it. Employers can play a crucial role in changing this by providing education and support for women in the workplace. This can include flexible working arrangements, access to counselling services and creating a culture of openness and understanding. By doing so, women can feel more comfortable and empowered to manage their symptoms and continue to thrive in their careers.

The Government Equalities Report on Menopause indicated that employers need to put in place training, processes and information so that *all* colleagues have a clear understanding of the menopause. The report suggested reasonable adjustments, such as desktop fans, extra uniforms and flexible working, all of which should be no more complicated to ask for than an ergonomic chair for your back. Menopause is now covered in the UK under the Equality Act 2010, which also deals with discrimination on the grounds of sex, age or disability.[52] I think it's good to know you have these rights because it isn't information that's widely shared.

This topic is juicy, and we are of a generation that is thankfully breaking our silence on it. Whispers of 'the change' are hopefully going to become roars from the once-invisible crew, no longer fading into the background but leading the way for the next generations to come. Intersectional layers of this are also worth nothing here – navigating help becomes more tricky if you are black or brown, trans or non-binary. I'm here to play my part in helping all aspects of care reach the people it needs to get to. This isn't going away, we aren't going away, hormones aren't going away – so, frankly, society, workplaces and the bloody patriarchy need to get with the programme and be cool. We all have a part to play in helping that to happen – let's get started.

CHAPTER 18 ROUND-UP

There is no right or wrong way to support yourself through YOUR menopause. But keep in mind that the following steps can help you:

- Preparing yourself for it ahead of the game
- Talking to others
- Researching and leaning in to how you would like to do it without feeling pressured into a camp
- Knowing there is a freedom that comes with the menopause and it's really time for you
- Communicating your needs to family friends and work
- Not feeling ashamed for going through a life stage – if you aren't being supported at work, you should be, and your employer has a duty of care to support you

Finally, don't suffer in silence. And feel safe in the knowledge you can now commit to wearing white pants till the end of time!

THE FINAL ROUND-UP

So, here we are at the end of the book. My hope for you is that you have learnt something, and that this has inspired, activated and empowered you, and that you feel confident in taking control of your own period and hormonal health now and forever, till death do you part! Share this book, pass it on to all the women and those who bleed. Everyone needs to know this stuff – it should be mainstream education.

When it comes to your health, question everything. Don't be agreeable just because you think someone is a professional. We are all humans at the end of the day, and it is important for you to feel like you are getting the best care. Pause as often as you need to, and don't be rushed into anything you aren't 100% comfortable with.

Remember: there is always more than one way to approach anything in life. Your route to helping yourself is your business. Opinions of others are like noses – we all have them, and they're generally best kept out of others' stuff. Just because people do things a different way doesn't make you wrong or right. If it works for you, then keep on rolling with it.

Always be aware of your energy – you only have a certain amount of fucks to give each day. Be mindful of how you use them; you might need to conserve some for another day. Or, go crazy and hand them out left right and centre. Only you know your capacity – don't go beyond it.

Remember your balance, but don't be scared of the face-plants because they are entirely necessary. You are a human being. I'm not asking for perfection from you, and neither should you be from yourself. The perfectly imperfect are my crew.

Finally, I want to say a massive thank you to my community and all the women I have worked with over the years. I have learnt so much from each of you. I have never tired of seeing you win, either; it fills my heart each time we unlock something that has been a mystery. Thank you for leaning in, being brave and taking the leap with me.

Go forth and be bloody amazing, walk with swagger, take no shit and above all else, put yourself at the top of that priority list... go on, I dare you.

Big love,
Gems x

THE WELL WOMAN PROJECT

If you have loved what you have read in this book and would like to learn more about how I work, you can find out about everything I offer, including my podcast, *Lost in Menstruation*, here: **www.thewellwomanproject.com**

To access the free charting course, visit:
www.thewellwomanproject.com/charting

Find my course "Unflappable: How Not to Lose Your Shit with Your Period" here:
www.thewellwomanproject.com/unflappable/

To listen to the meditation on page 190, visit:
www.thewellwomanproject.com/body-scan/

You can also follow The Well Woman Project on social media:

- **Facebook**: https://www.facebook.com/thewellwomanproject/
- **Instagram**: @well_woman_project
- **TikTok**: @well_woman_project

USEFUL RESOURCES

Here are a few more useful links that I tell my clients about and use/have used regularly myself:

- **thinkdirtyapp.com** – helps you to find out how clean your personal and household products are
- **earthwisegirls.co.uk** – for all variety of period product supplies
- **www.pogp.csp.org.uk** – a register of all qualified women's health physiotherapists in the UK; also contains information on pelvic floor dysfunction and other resources
- **www.vaginamuseum.co.uk** – a great place to spend a couple of hours in London
- **www.evolvebeauty.co.uk** – organic beauty products
- **zaoessenceofnature.co.uk** – more organic makeup and beauty products
- **www.theafrohairandskincompany.co.uk** – plant-based hair and skin care products
- **www.mygfbakery.com** – the best GF bagels I have found!

ACKNOWLEDGEMENTS

Thank you to my family – Mark, my hubby, for holding my hand, mopping my brow and the endless cups of tea. Indie, my heartbeat on four legs, you have no idea how grateful I am for all the walks. Rosie, my niece, for being your glorious self, the best shopping buddy and making me laugh.

My found family, Cath, Fran and Liz, thank you for all the shits and giggles. My Sov sisters, Cat M and Cat P, you have literally walked this with me! My witchy wild women, Afric, Bo, Juli, Nat, Rozi and Shelly, your love and support has meant the world. To all of you who have asked how the book is going, thank you for all the cheerleading, phone calls, meals out, tea, cake and laughter.

Thank you to my communities in comedy, Thrive, Sovereign and Wild Women, I would have been lost without you all. Your belief in me and The Well Woman Project has been unwavering. To all those that have helped me grow The Well Woman Project over the years, your mentoring, teachings, learnings and more have been invaluable.

Thank you to all those I have worked with at Trigger Publishing for giving me the opportunity to write this book.

Thank you to my wonderful, kick-ass clients and my online community who contribute to and share my work – you are the best. I am humbled and energised by you all!

Lastly, I want to thank myself, for digging deep and rising to the challenge. It's been a mountain, but I am so proud of myself. I won't lie, it feels weird to write a thank you to me, but also absolutely perfect and so very Snoop Dogg.

REFERENCES

1 Chai, S., & Wild, R. A. (1990). Basal body temperature and endometriosis. *Fertility and sterility*, 54(6), 1028–1031. https://doi.org/10.1016/s0015-0282(16)54000-x Knight, J. (2017). *The Complete Guide to Fertility Awareness* (pp. 217–217).

2 Routledge. Royal College of Obstetricians and Gynaecologists. (2022, April 4). More than half a million women face prolonged waits for gynaecology care. *RCOG*. https://www.rcog.org.uk/news/more-than-half-a-million-women-face-prolonged-waits-for-gynaecology-care/

3 Gregory, A. (2022, December 19). Tories 'failing women' as gynaecology waiting times treble in a decade. *The Guardian*. https://www.theguardian.com/society/2022/dec/19/tories-failing-women-as-gynaecology-waiting-times-treble-in-decade-nhs.

4 Simon, M. (2014, May 7). Fantastically wrong: The theory of the wandering wombs that drove women to madness. *Wired*. https://www.wired.com/2014/05/fantastically-wrong-wandering-womb/

5 Gilbert, S.F. (2000) Sex determination. *Developmental Biology, 6*. Sinaeur Associates. https://www.ncbi.nlm.nih.gov/books/NBK9985/

6 Culley, L., Law, C., Hudson, N., Mitchell, E., Denny, N. & Raine-Fenning, N. (2017, August). A qualitative study of the impact of endometriosis on male partners. *Human Reproduction*, 32(8), 1667–1673. https://doi.org/10.1093/humrep/dex221

7 Jackson, G. (2020, August 5). "Disgusting" study rating attractiveness of women with endometriosis retracted by Medical Journal. *The Guardian*. https://www.theguardian.com/society/2020/aug/05/disgusting-study-rating-attractiveness-of-women-with-endometriosis-retracted-by-medical-journal

8   Maserejian, N. N., Link, C. L., Lutfey, K. L., Marceau, L. D., &
     McKinlay, J. B. (2009). Disparities in Physicians' Interpretations of
     Heart Disease Symptoms by Patient Gender: Results of a Video
     Vignette Factorial Experiment. *Journal of Women's Health*,
     18(10), 1661-1667. https://doi.org/10.1089/jwh.2008.1007

9   Campbell, D. (2022) Women 32% more likely to die after
     operation by male surgeon, study reveals. *The Guardian*.
     https://www.theguardian.com/society/2022/jan/04/women-
     more-likely-die-operation-male-surgeon-study.

10   University of Miami. (2021, April 6). Women's pain not
     taken as seriously as men's pain: A new study suggests
     that when men and women express the same amount of
     pain, women's pain is considered less intense based on
     gender stereotypes. *ScienceDaily*. www.sciencedaily.com/
     releases/2021/04/210406164124.htm

11   Latifi, F. (2021, July 26). The Pain Gap: Why Women's Pain is
     Undertreated. *HealthyWomen*. https://www.healthywomen.
     org/condition/pain-gap-womens-pain-undertreated

12   Billock, J. (2018, May 22). *Pain bias: The health inequality rarely
     discussed*. https://www.bbc.com/future/article/20180518-the-
     inequality-in-how-women-are-treated-for-pain

13   Wind, R. (2011, November 15). Many American Women Use Birth
     Control Pills for Noncontraceptive Reasons. *Guttmacher Institute*.
     https://www.guttmacher.org/news-release/2011/many-american-
     women-use-birth-control-pills-noncontraceptive-reasons

14   Rutgers International (n.d.). Dutch Attitudes and Approaches
     to Sexuality. https://rutgers.international/about-rutgers/dutch-
     attitudes-and-approaches-to-sexuality/

15   Sedgh, G., Finer, L. B., Bankole, A., Eilers, M. A., & Singh,
     S. (2015). Adolescent Pregnancy, Birth, and Abortion Rates
     Across Countries: Levels and Recent Trends. *The Journal
     of Adolescent Health: Official Publication of the Society for
     Adolescent Medicine*, *56*(2), 223. https://doi.org/10.1016/j.
     jadohealth.2014.09.007

16   NHS (n.d.). *Drink Less.* NHS: Better Health, Let's Do This. https://
     www.nhs.uk/better-health/drink-less/#:~:text=Alcohol%20
     guidelines,risk%20of%20harming%20your%20health.

17   Marziali, M., Venza, M., Lazzaro, S., Lazzaro, A., Micossi,
     C., & Stolfi, V. M. (2012). Gluten-free diet: a new strategy
     for management of painful endometriosis related
     symptoms?. *Minerva chirurgica, 67*(6), 499–504.

18   World Health Organization (2021, May 1). *Replace: Trans Fat
     Free by 2023.* https://www.who.int/teams/nutrition-and-food-
     safety/replace-trans-fat

19   World Health Organization (2023, January 23). *Five billion
     people unprotected from trans fat leading to heart disease.*
     https://www.who.int/news/item/23-01-2023-five-billion-people-
     unprotected-from-trans-fat-leading-to-heart-disease

20   Willett, W. C., & Ascherio, A. (1994) Trans fatty acids: are
     the effects only marginal?. *American Journal of Public
     Health 84,* 722–724, https://doi.org/10.2105/AJPH.84.5.722

21   Keendjele, T. P. T., Eelu, H. H., Nashihanga, T. E., Rennie,
     T. W., & Hunter, C. J. (2021). Corn? When did I eat corn?
     Gastrointestinal transit time in health science students.
     Advances in Psychology Education, 45(1), 103–108. https://doi.
     org/10.1152/advan.00192.2020

22   Sweney, M. (2022, August 12). Johnson & Johnson to stop
     making talc-based baby powder globally. *The Guardian.*
     https://www.theguardian.com/business/2022/aug/12/johnson-
     and-johnson-to-stop-making-talc-based-baby-powder-globally

23   Chang, C. J., O'Brien, K. M., Keil, A. P., Gaston, S. A., Jackson,
     C. L., Sandler, D. P., & White, A. J. (2022). Use of Straighteners
     and Other Hair Products and Incident Uterine Cancer. *Journal
     of the National Cancer Institute, 114*(12), 1636–1645. https://
     doi.org/10.1093/jnci/djac165

24   Suliman, A. (2022, October 18). Johnson & Johnson to stop
     making talc-based baby powder globally. *The Washington
     Post.* https://www.washingtonpost.com/health/2022/10/18/
     chemical-hair-straightening-uterine-cancer-black-women-nih/

25 Perkins, T. (2022, September 23). 'Forever chemicals' detected in all umbilical cord blood in 40 studies. *The Guardian.* https://www.theguardian.com/environment/2022/sep/23/forever-chemicals-found-umbilical-cord-blood-samples-studies

26 Perkins, T. (2022, October 5). Study links in utero 'forever chemical' exposure to low sperm count and mobility. *The Guardian.* https://www.theguardian.com/society/2022/oct/05/pfas-sperm-count-mobility-testicle-development

27 Niema, D. C., & Wentz, L. M. (2019). The compelling link between physical activity and the body's defense system. *Journal of Sport and Health Science, 8*(3), 201-217. https://doi.org/10.1016/j.jshs.2018.09.009

28 Gladwell, V. F., Brown, D. K., Wood, C., Sandercock, G. R., & Barton, J. L. (2013). The great outdoors: how a green exercise environment can benefit all. *Extreme physiology & medicine, 2*(1), 3. https://doi.org/10.1186/2046-7648-2-3

29 Kennedy, G., Hardman, R. J., Macpherson, H., Scholey, A. B., & Pipingas, A. (2017). How Does Exercise Reduce the Rate of Age-Associated Cognitive Decline? A Review of Potential Mechanisms. *Journal of Alzheimer's Disease, 55*(1), 1-18. https://doi.org/10.3233/JAD-160665

30 Encyclopædia Brittanica (n.d.). *Stress Definition & Meaning.* The Britannica Dictionary. https://www.britannica.com/dictionary/stress

31 Turakitwanakan, W., Mekseepralard, C., & Busarakumtragul, P. (2013). Effects of mindfulness meditation on serum cortisol of medical students. *Journal of the Medical Association of Thailand = Chotmaihet thangphaet, 96*(1), S90–S95.

32 Thatcher, L. (2021, March 29). *Millican's Law for Preachers.* Liam Thatcher. https://liamthatcher.com/2021/03/29/millicans-law-for-preachers/#:~:text=Sarah%20says%20this%2C,it%20and%20forget%20about%20it

33 Azzazy, S., Ghaffarianhoseini, A., Hoseini, A. G., Naismith, N. & Doborjeh, Z. (2021). A critical review on the impact of built environment on users' measured brain activity, *Architectural*

Science Review, 64(4), 319-335, https://doi.org/10.1080/00038
628.2020.1749980

34   Brown, L. (1994). Live Your Dreams (p. 194). William Morrow.

35   Patrick, M., MD (2022, May 16). Spending Time Outdoors
Promotes Good Mental Health. Nationwide Children's.
https://www.nationwidechildrens.org/family-resources-
education/700childrens/2022/05/spending-time-outdoors-
promotes-good-mental-health

36   Day, A. (2023, May 26). 'It's easier to get a condom than a pad':
Lacking period products, a third of girls miss school. INews.
https://inews.co.uk/news/health/lacking-period-products-girls-
miss-school-2366152

37   HM Treasury (2021, January 1). Tampon tax abolished from
today. https://www.gov.uk/government/news/tampon-tax-
abolished-from-today

38   Phillips, T. (2016, August 16). 'It's because I had my period':
Swimmer Fu Yuanhui praised for breaking taboo. The Guardian.
https://www.theguardian.com/sport/2016/aug/16/chinese-
swimmer-fu-yuanhui-praised-for-breaking-periods-taboo

39   Ingle, S. (2022, August 19). Dina Asher-Smith praised for shattering
'massive taboo' around periods in sport. The Guardian. https://
www.theguardian.com/sport/2022/aug/19/dina-asher-smith-
praised-for-shattering-massive-taboo-around-periods-in-sport

40   (2022, February 1). Menopause. Menopause and Me. https://
www.menopauseandme.co.uk/en-gb/menopause-and-me/
stages-and-symptoms-of-menopause/menopause

41   (2022, February 1). Menopause. Menopause and Me. https://
www.menopauseandme.co.uk/en-gb/menopause-and-me/
stages-and-symptoms-of-menopause/menopause

42   Tucci, J. R. (2008). Importance of Early Diagnosis and
Treatment of Osteoporosis to Prevent Fractures. American
Journal of Managed Care, 12(7 Suppl), 181-190. https://www.
ajmc.com/view/may06-2313ps181-s190

43   (2019, August 15). Know Your Osteoporosis Risk. Healthline.
https://www.healthline.com/health/osteoporosis-risk-factors

44   Salari, P., & Abdollahi, M. (2014). The influence of pregnancy and lactation on maternal bone health: a systematic review. *Journal of family & reproductive health, 8*(4), 135–148.

45   Leyland, S. (2021, March 22). *What's the menopause got to do with bone health?* Royal Osteoporosis Society. https://theros.org.uk/blog/2021-03-22-what-s-the-menopause-got-to-do-with-bone-health

46   Alzheimer's Society. (n.d.). *Hormones and dementia.* https://www.alzheimers.org.uk/about-dementia/risk-factors-and-prevention/hormones-and-dementia

47   British Menopause Society (2020, July 9). *Possible link between hormones and Alzheimer's Dementia.* https://thebms.org.uk/2020/07/possible-link-between-hormones-and-alzheimers-dementia/

48   Koblinsky, N. D., Meusel, L. C., Greenwood, C. E., & Anderson, N. D. (2021). Household physical activity is positively associated with gray matter volume in older adults. *BMC Geriatrics, 21.* https://doi.org/10.1186/s12877-021-02054-8

49   British Heart Foundation (n.d.). *Menopause and Heart Disease.* https://www.bhf.org.uk/informationsupport/support/women-with-a-heart-condition/menopause-and-heart-disease

50   Grand View Research (n.d.). *Menopause Market Size, Share & Trends Analysis Report By Treatment.* https://www.grandviewresearch.com/industry-analysis/menopause-market

51   Women's Health Concern (n.d.). *Menopause in the Workplace.* https://www.womens-health-concern.org/help-and-advice/menopause-in-the-workplace/

52   Department for Work & Pensions (2022, July 18). *Menopause and the Workplace: How to enable fulfilling working lives: Government response.* https://www.gov.uk/government/publications/menopause-and-the-workplace-how-to-enable-fulfilling-working-lives-government-response/menopause-and-the-workplace-how-to-enable-fulfilling-working-lives-government-response

TriggerHub.org is one of the most elite and scientifically proven forms of mental health intervention

Trigger Publishing is the leading independent mental health and wellbeing publisher in the UK and US. Our collection of bibliotherapeutic books and the power of lived experience changes lives forever. Our courageous authors' lived experiences and the power of their stories are scientifically endorsed by independent federal, state and privately funded research in the US. These stories are intrinsic elements in reducing stigma, making those with poor mental health feel less alone, giving them the privacy they need to heal, ensuring they are guided by the essential steps to kick-start their own journeys to recovery, and providing hope and inspiration when they need it most.

Clinical and scientific research conducted by assistant professor Dr Kristin Kosyluk and her highly acclaimed team in the Department of Mental Health Law & Policy at the University of South Florida (USF), as well as complementary research by her peers across the US, has independently verified the power of lived experience as a core component in achieving mental health prosperity. Their findings categorically confirm lived experience as a leading method in treating those struggling with poor mental health by significantly reducing stigma and the time it takes for them to seek help, self-help or signposting if they are struggling.

Delivered through TriggerHub, our unique online portal and smartphone app, we make our library of bibliotherapeutic titles and other vital resources accessible to individuals and organizations anywhere, at any time and with complete privacy, a crucial element of recovery. As such, TriggerHub is the primary recommendation across the UK and US for the delivery of lived experiences.

Technology will, of course, always evolve, come and go. But the practice of prescribing books for guidance and healing has been around since the Middle Ages – the word bibliotherapy is a combination of the Greek words for "book" and "healing". TriggerHub combines this steadfast practice with our world-renowned, scientifically backed USP and powerful stories from our authors, thus creating the blueprint for delivering lived experiences, making mental health recovery possible and instilling the key components of mental health prosperity in today's generation – and generations to come.

At Trigger Publishing and TriggerHub, we proudly lead the way in making the unseen become seen. We are dedicated to humanizing mental health, breaking stigma and challenging outdated societal values to create real action and impact. Find out more about our world-leading work with lived experience and bibliotherapy via triggerhub.org, or by joining us on:

𝕏 @triggerhub_

f @triggerhub.org

◎ @triggerhub_

Dr Kristin Kosyluk, Ph.D., is an assistant professor in the Department of Mental Health Law and Policy at USF, a faculty affiliate of the Louis de la Parte Florida Mental Health Institute, and director of the STigma Action Research (STAR) Lab. Find out more about Dr Kristin Kosyluk, her team and their work by visiting:

USF Department of Mental Health Law & Policy:
www.usf.edu/cbcs/mhlp/index.aspx

USF College of Behavioral and Community Sciences:
www.usf.edu/cbcs/index.aspx

STAR Lab: www.usf.edu/cbcs/mhlp/centers/star-lab/

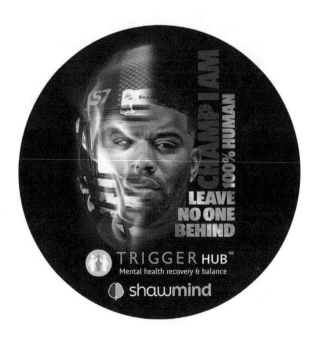

CHAMP I AM 100% HUMAN

LEAVE NO ONE BEHIND

TRIGGER HUB™
Mental health recovery & balance

shawmind

For more information, visit BJ-Super7.com

Printed in the USA
CPSIA information can be obtained
at www.ICGtesting.com
JSHW010321111123
51877JS00004B/9